Florida MPJE® Exam Prep

300 Pharmacy Law Practice Questions

- ☑ 100 FEDERAL LAW QUESTIONS
- ☑ 200 FLORIDA LAW QUESTIONS

PHARMACY TESTING SOLUTIONS

SECOND EDITION: REVISED FOR 2025

ISBN: 979-8-3741-2496-5

Table of Contents

Introduction

The Multistate Pharmacy Jurisprudence Examination (MPJE) is a pharmacy law exam developed by the National Association of Boards of Pharmacy (NABP). It assesses candidates' knowledge and competency in pharmacy law. The exam comprises 120 questions, combining federal and state-specific content, covering four content areas: Licensure/Personnel (22%); Pharmacist Practice (33%); Dispensing Requirements (24%); and Pharmacy Operations (21%).

This book is designed to help you prepare for both federal and state questions across all content areas. The first section presents 100 questions on federal pharmacy law, while the second section offers 200 questions on Florida state pharmacy law. An answer index with detailed explanations for each question is provided at the back of the book. When taking the MPJE, it's crucial to select the stricter law when discrepancies exist between federal and state regulations.

When preparing for the MPJE, focus fully, read each question carefully, and aim to simulate exam conditions by working through your practice questions without interruptions. The actual exam is 2.5 hours long, so it may be beneficial to time yourself during practice sessions to ensure you're allocating an appropriate amount of time to each question.

On the day of the exam, ensure you're well-rested, eat a substantial breakfast, and arrive at the testing center at least 30 minutes early for check-in procedures. Bring one valid, government-issued photo ID that includes a recognizable photograph and your signature, as this is required for admission to the testing center.

Good luck with the MPJE, and happy studying!

Federal MPJE Practice Questions

1. What was the first law requiring drugs to be proven safe before being marketed?
   a. Food, Drug, and Cosmetic Act
   b. Kefauver-Harris Amendment
   c. Pure Food and Drug Act
   d. Prescription Drug Marketing Act
   e. Durham-Humphrey Amendment

2. A pharmacist receives an urgent notification from a manufacturing company for a recall of a specific medication because it may cause serious adverse health issues or death. What type of drug recall is this?
   a. Class I
   b. Class II
   c. Class III
   d. Class IV
   e. Class V

3. What agency is responsible for the federal Controlled Substances Act (CSA)?
   a. Federal Bureau of Investigation (FBI)
   b. Food and Drug Administration (FDA)
   c. Department of Health and Human Services (HHS)
   d. Drug Enforcement Administration (DEA)
   e. United States Pharmacopeia (USP)

4. A pharmacist wants to know if generic warfarin tablets are bioequivalent to brand name Coumadin tablets. Where can this information be found?
    a. The Purple Book
    b. The Blue Book
    c. The Green Book
    d. The Orange Book
    e. The Red Book

5. Which of the following is NOT required on the manufacturer's drug container label for an oral drug product?
    a. Name of the manufacturer
    b. Expiration date
    c. Name of the drug or product
    d. Directions for administration
    e. Net quantity packaged

6. According to federal law, what age must the purchaser be to purchase a controlled substance without a prescription that contains opium?
    a. 16
    b. 18
    c. 21
    d. 25
    e. No age requirement

7. Which DEA form must be completed and submitted to the DEA upon discovering a theft or significant loss of controlled substances?
    a. DEA Form 106
    b. DEA Form 108
    c. DEA Form 222
    d. DEA Form 224
    e. DEA Form 363

8. Which of the following is a Schedule II controlled substance?
    a. Buprenorphine
    b. Butabarbital
    c. Mescaline
    d. Pentobarbital
    e. Modafinil

9. A non-preserved aqueous oral formulation that is compounded from commercially available drug products has a maximum beyond-use date (BUD) of _____ when refrigerated.
   a. 3 days
   b. 7 days
   c. 14 days
   d. 30 days
   e. 45 days

10. Practitioners who dispense methadone for detoxification must register for a narcotic treatment program using what form?
    a. DEA Form 222
    b. DEA Form 224
    c. DEA Form 363
    d. DEA Form 106
    e. DEA Form 41

11. Which FDA expedited review program is intended for drugs that treat serious conditions and fill an unmet medical need?
    a. Breakthrough therapy
    b. Instant approval
    c. Fast track
    d. Accelerated approval
    e. Priority review

12. Schedule II controlled substances CANNOT be transferred in which of the following scenarios?
    a. A pharmacy is closing and decides to transfer their Schedule II controlled substance inventory to another pharmacy
    b. A pharmacy is not renewing their DEA registration and therefore wants to transfer their remaining Schedule II controlled substances to another pharmacy
    c. A pharmacy ordered the wrong Schedule II controlled substances and wants to transfer them back to the supplier
    d. A researcher would like to transfer excess Schedule II controlled substances to a pharmacy to be dispensed to patients
    e. A pharmacy wants to transfer 2 bottles of Schedule II controlled substances to another pharmacy

13. A patient wants to refill a prescription but was not satisfied with the pharmacy that filled and dispensed the prescription the first time. The patient demands the prescription be returned so they can take it to a different pharmacy to obtain refills. The pharmacist should:
    a. Document the original fill information on the original prescription, keep a copy, and return the original prescription to the patient
    b. Offer to give a copy of the prescription to the patient, keep the original copy at the pharmacy, and recommend the patient request the prescription be transferred to another pharmacy if legal
    c. Void the original prescription before returning it to the patient and offer to transfer the rest verbally to another pharmacy
    d. Document the situation in the patient's profile and return the original prescription to the patient
    e. Inform the patient you can send the prescription by priority mail to the pharmacy of their choice

14. When a pharmacy submits a DEA Form 222 (single sheet) to purchase Schedule II controlled substances, who keeps the original copy of the DEA Form 222?
    a. The pharmacy
    b. The supplier
    c. The manufacturer
    d. The DEA
    e. The pharmacist

15. For which type of drug recall is there a possibility of temporary or medically reversible adverse effects, but the probability of serious adverse effects is remote?
    a. Class I
    b. Class II
    c. Class III
    d. Class A
    e. Class B

16. A drug has an NDC of 16103-0350-11. The 0350 represents:
    a. The manufacturer name
    b. The amount packaged
    c. The identity of the drug
    d. The location of manufacturing
    e. The route of administration

17. What set of regulations specifies the required minimum manufacturing standards for pharmaceutical products in the U.S.?
    a. Standards of Manufacturing Practice (SMP)
    b. Good Pharmaceutical Manufacturing Practice (GPMP)
    c. Requirements of Good Manufacturing Practice (RGMP)
    d. Regulations of Manufacturing Practice (RMP)
    e. Good Manufacturing Practice (GMP)

18. A prescriber may issue multiple prescriptions authorizing a patient to receive a total of up to a 90-day supply of a Schedule II controlled substance if certain conditions are met. Which of the following is NOT one of those conditions?
    a. Each separate prescription must be issued for a legitimate medical purpose
    b. The prescriber must include written instructions on each consecutive prescription indicating the earliest month in which a pharmacy may fill it
    c. The prescriber must conclude that providing the patient with multiple prescriptions will not create an undue risk of diversion or abuse
    d. The issuance of multiple prescriptions must be permissible under the applicable state law
    e. The prescriber must comply fully with all other applicable requirements

19. A prescription for lorazepam can be refilled a maximum of how many times within a six-month period?
    a. Zero
    b. Two
    c. Three
    d. Five
    e. Six

20. In order for buprenorphine to be prescribed, which of the following conditions must be met?
    a. The prescriber's liability insurance must provide buprenorphine indemnity
    b. The prescriber must have less than 30 patients to whom they prescribe buprenorphine
    c. The prescriber must have been granted a waiver from the DEA in order to prescribe buprenorphine
    d. The prescriber must have an active DEA license that includes the schedule in which buprenorphine is listed
    e. The prescriber must have an active "X" number

21. An example of an adulterated drug is:
    a. The name of the manufacturer is not included on the label
    b. A medication that has an unapproved color additive
    c. Active ingredients are missing from the bottle
    d. The drug causes an allergic reaction in the patient
    e. The drug container does not contain proper directions for nonprescription drugs

22. Which of the following is a mid-level practitioner?
    a. Physician
    b. Dentist
    c. Veterinarian
    d. Optometrist
    e. Podiatrist

23. Durable Medical Equipment (DME) must meet which standard(s)? Select ALL that apply.
    a. Can withstand repeated use
    b. Strictly for assistance with walking
    c. Limited to use for paraplegics
    d. Appropriate for use in the home
    e. Primarily for a medical purpose

24. What act regulates the sale and recordkeeping requirements for prescription drug samples?
    a. Prescription Drug Marketing Act
    b. Durham–Humphrey Amendment
    c. Pure Food and Drug Act
    d. Food, Drug and Cosmetic Act
    e. Kefauver-Harris Amendment

25. Which of the following can be determined from the National Drug Code (NDC) number on a medication bottle? Select ALL that apply.
    a. Manufacturer
    b. Specific drug
    c. Package
    d. Expiration date
    e. FDA approval status

26. Under the iPLEDGE Risk Evaluation and Mitigation Strategy (REMS) for isotretinoin, what is the maximum number of refills that may be authorized on a prescription?
    a. 0 refills
    b. 1 refill
    c. 2 refills
    d. 5 refills
    e. 11 refills

27. In which situation would it be illegal for a pharmacy to compound drugs?
    a. The quantity prepared is reasonable for filling existing and anticipated prescriptions
    b. Dosage forms are sold only to other pharmacies and not physician offices
    c. Ingredients in the compounded drugs meet national standards
    d. The compounded drug is not commercially available
    e. Interstate distribution of compounded drugs is no more than 5% of total prescriptions sold by the pharmacy per year

28. What DEA form is necessary to purchase or transfer Schedule II controlled substances?
    a. DEA Form 108
    b. DEA Form 222
    c. DEA Form 224
    d. DEA Form 225
    e. DEA Form 363

29. A patient calls the pharmacy and says they just got home from the hospital after having broken their leg. The patient cannot make it to the pharmacy to pick up their prescription for a Schedule II controlled substance that is ready to pick up. The patient asks if the pharmacy can mail the prescription to the house (mail delivery). How should the pharmacist respond?
    a. Controlled substance medications cannot be mailed
    b. Only Schedule III–V controlled substances can be mailed
    c. Controlled substances can only be mailed to the prescriber's office for office pickup
    d. The prescription can be sent to the patient through the mail
    e. The prescription can be sent to the patient as long as the drug name is listed on the package

30. Which of the following statements is/are true about narrow therapeutic index (NTI) drugs?

    I. Small differences in the dose or blood concentration may lead to adverse reactions

    II. They are not permitted to be prescribed

    III. They require careful titration or patient monitoring for safe and effective use

    a. I only
    b. II only
    c. I and III only
    d. II and III only
    e. I, II, and III

31. What act set the requirement for child-resistant closures for prescription drugs, non-prescription drugs, and hazardous household products?
    a. Poison Prevention Packaging Act
    b. Child Drug Safety Act
    c. Prevention of Hazardous Consumption Act
    d. Children Poison Prevention Act
    e. Hazardous Materials Safety Act

32. According to the Combat Methamphetamine Epidemic Act of 2005, the logbook requirement does NOT apply to individual single sales of packages of:
    a. No more than 60mg of pseudoephedrine
    b. No less than 60mg of pseudoephedrine
    c. No more than 50mg of pseudoephedrine
    d. No less than 50mg of pseudoephedrine
    e. All pseudoephedrine sales are required to be logged

33. Over-the-counter (OTC) drug advertising is regulated by the:
    a. Federal Trade Commission
    b. Food and Drug Administration
    c. Drug Quality and Security Commission
    d. Consumer Product Safety Commission
    e. None of the above

34. What information is required to be included in the transaction report transmitted from a manufacturer to a pharmacy when the pharmacy purchases bulk bottles of a medication?
    a. Transaction information, transaction history, transaction log
    b. Transaction purpose, transaction history, transaction ID number
    c. Transaction information, transaction history, transaction statement
    d. Transaction ID number, transaction code, transaction statement
    e. Transaction purpose, transaction history, transaction log

35. What law requires drugs to be proven effective (as well as safe) before being marketed?
    a. Durham-Humphrey Amendment
    b. Pure Food and Drug Act
    c. Prescription Drug Marketing Act
    d. Hatch-Waxman Amendment
    e. Kefauver-Harris Amendment

36. Which DEA registration form is used for pharmacies to register with the DEA to possess and dispense controlled substances?
    a. DEA Form 106
    b. DEA Form 222
    c. DEA Form 224
    d. DEA Form 225
    e. DEA Form 363

37. Re-importation of medications is only legal if performed by the:

    I.   Retail pharmacy

    II. Original manufacturer

    III. Wholesale distributor

    a. I only
    b. II only
    c. III only
    d. I and III only
    e. I, II, and III

38. Which of the following is true regarding the stocking and dispensing of methadone at retail pharmacies?
    a. Methadone may not be stocked or dispensed from a retail pharmacy; patients must obtain methadone from a narcotic treatment facility
    b. Methadone may be stocked at a retail pharmacy, but may only be dispensed as an analgesic
    c. Methadone may be stocked at a retail pharmacy, but may only be dispensed for narcotic dependence
    d. Methadone may be stocked at a retail pharmacy and may be dispensed as either an analgesic or for the short-term treatment of narcotic dependence
    e. Methadone may be stocked at any pharmacy and may be dispensed as either an analgesic or for the long-term treatment of narcotic dependence

39. What act requires health care facilities to report death or injuries caused by or suspected to have been caused by a medical device to the FDA or the manufacturer?
    a. FDA Modernization Act
    b. Medical Device Inspection Act
    c. Safe Medical Device Act
    d. Pure Food and Drug Act
    e. The Omnibus Budget Reconciliation Act

40. An example of a misbranded manufacturer's container of a drug would be:
    a. The drug causes an allergic reaction in the patient
    b. The container is made of a substance that leaches into the medication
    c. There is no quantity of the contents listed on the container
    d. The drug is exposed to unsanitary conditions
    e. The patient writes the indication for the medication on their prescription bottle

41. Which of the following requirements must be met for a controlled substance prescription to be valid? Select ALL that apply.
    a. Must be manually signed if it is a paper or faxed prescription
    b. Must be issued for a legitimate medical purpose
    c. Must be prescribed in the usual course of medical treatment
    d. Must be issued to an individual practitioner for the purpose of general dispensing to patients
    e. Must be dated and signed on the fill date

42. According to the FDA, a drug is considered to be an orphan drug if it is for rare diseases or conditions that impact fewer than how many people in the U.S.?
    a. 10
    b. 500
    c. 200,000
    d. 1,000,000
    e. 2,000,000

43. Which of the following ingredients has special labeling requirements if it is included in a product?
    a. Gelatin
    b. FD&C Yellow No. 5
    c. High fructose corn syrup
    d. Sorbitol
    e. Xanthan gum

44. In which case(s) is it appropriate to receive a faxed prescription for a Schedule II controlled substance?

    I. Patient is a resident of a long-term care facility (LTCF)

    II. Patient is enrolled in hospice program

    III. Medication is intended for home infusion therapy

    a. I only
    b. II only
    c. I and II
    d. II and III
    e. I, II, and III

45. What is the acronym of the voluntary reporting system for medication adverse events?
    a. VAERS
    b. FAERS
    c. ERSA
    d. MAERS
    e. AERS

46. Within how many days must a prescriber deliver a written prescription for a Schedule II controlled substance that was called in orally to be dispensed in an emergency situation?
    a. 3 days
    b. 5 days
    c. 7 days
    d. 14 days
    e. 15 days

47. A pharmacy intern wants to know where to find information on therapeutic equivalence between biologics. Which book contains this information?
    a. Red Book
    b. Purple Book
    c. Pink Book
    d. Orange Book
    e. Yellow Book

48. In which case(s) must an exact count be taken while performing a controlled substance inventory?

    I.   It is a Schedule II controlled substance

    II. The bottle holds more than 1000 tablets or capsules

    III. Containers are sealed or unopened

    a. I only
    b. II only
    c. I and II
    d. II and III
    e. I, II, and III

49. The scheduling of controlled substances at the federal level is performed by the:
    a. Food and Drug Administration
    b. U.S. Attorney General
    c. Drug Enforcement Agency
    d. National Board of Pharmacy
    e. Drug Enforcement Administration

50. A manufacturer of a prescription-only drug wants to reclassify the drug as an over-the-counter (OTC) drug. What is one of the forms that may be submitted to the FDA when requesting reclassification of a prescription-only drug to an over-the-counter drug?
    a. Emergency Investigational New Drug Application (EIND)
    b. Investigational New Drug Application (IND)
    c. New Drug Application (NDA)
    d. Abbreviated New Drug Application (ANDA)
    e. Marketed New Drug Application (MNDA)

51. You are a pharmacist that suspects a fake controlled substance prescription was called in to your pharmacy. You use the numbers in the provided DEA to verify if it is a true DEA number. It is indeed not a true DEA number because the last number is incorrect. The DEA number is BS5927683. What would be the correct last digit of the DEA number if it was accurate?
    a. 1
    b. 2
    c. 4
    d. 5
    e. 6

52. Which of the following prescriptions would likely be out of the scope of practice for a dentist?
    a. Tylenol #3
    b. Amoxicillin
    c. Lorazepam
    d. Atorvastatin
    e. None of the above; dentists are not limited to scope of practice

53. Who is authorized to sign a DEA Form 222 at a community pharmacy?
    a. Any pharmacist
    b. Any pharmacist or technician
    c. Only the pharmacist-in-charge
    d. Only the pharmacist who signed the most recent application for renewal of the pharmacy's DEA registration
    e. The pharmacist who signed the most recent application for renewal of the pharmacy's DEA registration or someone authorized under a power of attorney

54. What types of patients are included in a Phase I clinical trial for drug development?
    a. Large group of non-human animals
    b. Small group of healthy participants without the disease condition
    c. Small group of participants with the disease condition
    d. Large group of healthy participants without the disease condition
    e. Large group of participants with the disease condition

55. A pharmacy may keep which of the following records at a central location other than the location registered with the DEA?
    a. Controlled substance inventories
    b. Controlled substance prescriptions
    c. Controlled substance shipping and financial records
    d. Copies of executed DEA Form 222 orders
    e. None of the above may be kept at a central location; all must be kept at the pharmacy

56. Acetaminophen with codeine (Tylenol #3) is classified under which controlled substance schedule?
    a. Schedule I
    b. Schedule II
    c. Schedule III
    d. Schedule IV
    e. Schedule V

57. A patient is admitted to a hospital and does not remember the names of the medications that she takes at home. The hospital pharmacist calls the patient's outpatient pharmacy to obtain a list of medications. Which of the following statements is true?
    a. This is a HIPAA violation unless the patient has given signed consent for the information to be given to the hospital
    b. This is a HIPAA violation unless the patient has given verbal consent for the information to be given to the hospital
    c. This is a HIPAA violation unless the patient has given written and verbal consent for the information to be given to the hospital
    d. This is not a HIPAA violation because HIPAA does not apply to patients being treated in a hospital setting
    e. This is not a HIPAA violation because the information is being given to the hospital for treatment purposes

58. A warning stating "Caution: Federal law prohibits the transfer of this drug to any person other than the patient for whom it was prescribed" is required on the label on which of the following prescriptions?
    a. Schedule II controlled substances only
    b. Schedule II–IV controlled substances only
    c. Schedule II–V controlled substances only
    d. Schedule III–V controlled substances only
    e. All prescriptions require this warning under federal law

59. Registering with the FDA as an outsourcing facility allows a pharmacy to:
    a. Compound sterile products without receiving patient-specific prescriptions
    b. Act as a mail order pharmacy with the ability to send medications to multiple states
    c. Process prescriptions and medication orders remotely for another pharmacy, but not dispense any medications
    d. Repackage medications so that they can be used at hospitals and other institutions
    e. Order drug products listed on the FDA drug shortage list at a discounted cost

60. In the event of a breach of unsecured protected health information (PHI) at a retail pharmacy affecting approximately 900 patients, who must be notified? Select ALL that apply.
    a. All nearby pharmacies
    b. Prominent local media outlets
    c. Affected patients
    d. All patients who use the pharmacy
    e. U.S. Secretary of Health and Human Services (HHS)

61. Standards and requirements for preparing sterile compounded drugs to ensure patient benefit and reduce risks such as contamination, infection, or incorrect dosing are outlined in which of the following?
    a. USP Chapter <503A>
    b. USP Chapter <503B>
    c. USP Chapter <795>
    d. USP Chapter <797>
    e. USP Chapter <800>

62. Which of the following is/are required to register with the Drug Enforcement Administration (DEA)? Select ALL that apply.
    a. A patient who receives a prescription for a controlled substance
    b. A manufacturer that manufactures controlled substances
    c. A pharmacy that dispenses controlled substances
    d. A physician who prescribes controlled substances
    e. A pharmacist who dispenses controlled substances

63. Which of the following medications requires Risk Evaluation and Mitigation Strategy (REMS) monitoring?
    a. Hydromorphone (Dilaudid)
    b. Clozapine (Clozaril)
    c. Fluoxetine (Prozac)
    d. Zolpidem (Ambien)
    e. Metformin (Glucophage)

64. A DEA Form 41 is used to document which of the following?
    a. Purchasing of controlled substances from a manufacturer
    b. Transfer of controlled substances to a reverse distributor
    c. On-site destruction of controlled substances
    d. Significant loss or theft of controlled substances
    e. None of the above

65. What act set the requirement for tamper-evident packaging for some over-the-counter products in order to avoid risk of contamination?
    a. Safe Drug Packaging Act
    b. Federal Anti-Tampering Act
    c. Drug Contamination Prevention Act
    d. Federal Anti-Contamination Act
    e. Tamper-Evident Packaging Act

66. Drugs that have a high potential for abuse and severe potential for dependence with no currently accepted medical use in the U.S. are classified as:
    a. Schedule I
    b. Schedule II
    c. Schedule III
    d. Schedule IV
    e. None of the above

67. Which of the following is NOT required to be included on a manufacturer's container of an over-the-counter (OTC) medication?
    a. Warnings
    b. Inactive ingredients
    c. Poison Control Center phone number
    d. Purpose
    e. Directions

68. A nursing home patient who is prescribed an estrogen-containing product must be given a Patient Package Insert (PPI):
    a. Prior to the first administration only
    b. Prior to the first administration and every 30 days thereafter
    c. Prior to the first administration and every 60 days thereafter
    d. Only when requested by the patient
    e. None of the above

69. For how long is a DEA registration for possession of controlled substances valid?
    a. 12 months
    b. 24 months
    c. 36 months
    d. 48 months
    e. 60 months

70. Which of the following statements is/are true regarding DEA Form 222?

    I.   Executed copies of DEA Form 222 must be maintained separately from all other records.

    II. A defective DEA Form 222 may be corrected and reused.

    III. On the DEA Form 222, only 1 item may be entered on each numbered line.

    a. I only
    b. II only
    c. I and III only
    d. II and III only
    e. I, II, and III

71. An independent community pharmacy wants to start offering refill reminders to patients in the form of a postcard mailed to the patient's house. The fee for this service would be $2 per month. Which of the following is true regarding this service?
    a. This service cannot be provided because it creates a HIPAA violation
    b. Signed authorization would be required from each patient, as this is considered use of protected health information (PHI) for marketing purposes
    c. This service does not violate HIPAA, but patients cannot be charged a fee for refill reminders
    d. This service does not violate HIPAA, but the reminders must be transmitted electronically
    e. There are no barriers to offering this service and the pharmacy can proceed as planned

72. The expiration date on a bottle of metformin purchased from a manufacturer by a pharmacy is listed as 03/22. What is the expiration date of the drug?
    a. March 1, 2022
    b. March 19, 2022
    c. March 30, 2022
    d. March 31, 2022
    e. None of the above

73. A prospective drug utilization review (DUR) consists of reviewing all of the following aspects of a prescription EXCEPT for:
    a. Underutilization
    b. Therapeutic duplication
    c. Compliance with prescription labeling
    d. Appropriate dosing and regimen
    e. Drug interactions

74. Which of the following statements is required on an over-the-counter (OTC) package of acetaminophen tablets under the Federal Hazardous Substances Act?
    a. "Keep out of the reach of children"
    b. "Consult a doctor before use"
    c. "Do not use if pregnant or breastfeeding"
    d. "Prescription not required"
    e. "For adult use only"

75. A pharmacy dispenses and distributes a total of 50,000 doses of controlled substances in a 12-month period. How many doses is the pharmacy able to transfer to another pharmacy without registering as a distributor?
    a. 500 doses
    b. 1,000 doses
    c. 2,500 doses
    d. 5,000 doses
    e. 10,000 doses

76. The Occupational and Safety Health Administration (OSHA) requires that pharmacies do which of the following?
    a. Provide patients with information regarding the safe handling of hazardous medications
    b. Provide patients with Safety Data Sheets for hazardous medications
    c. Include the word "caution" or "warning" on labels for all hazardous medications
    d. Train all of their employees on the hazards of chemicals and on the protective measures they should take
    e. None of the above

77. The Poison Prevention Packaging Act (PPPA), which requires child-resistant containers for prescription and certain non-prescription drugs (with some exceptions), is administered by the:
    a. Food and Drug Administration
    b. Consumer Product Safety Commission
    c. Federal Trade Commission
    d. Centers for Medicare and Medicaid Services
    e. Occupational and Safety Health Administration

78. A pharmacy orders bulk bottles of ibuprofen and compounds ibuprofen suppositories. These suppositories are sold to other pharmacies that need to fill prescriptions but do not have the ability to make them. Which of the following terms best describes this practice?
    a. Compounding
    b. Dispensing
    c. Bulk compounding
    d. Manufacturing
    e. Outsourcing

79. Which of the following is true regarding the purchasing and selling of prescription drug samples?
    a. Drug samples may be purchased by a community pharmacy from a drug company and sold to patients at a standard price set by the FDA
    b. Drug samples may be purchased by a community pharmacy but must be given to patients free of charge
    c. Drug samples may only be given to a patient at a community pharmacy if the patient already has a prescription for the same medication
    d. Drug samples may be given to a pharmacy owned by a charitable organization and sold to patients at a reduced cost if the facility provides care to indigent or low-income patients
    e. Drug samples may be given to a pharmacy which is owned by a charitable organization that provides care to indigent or low-income patients, but must be given to patients free of charge

80. Which of the following is a valid method of ordering Schedule III medications from a supplier to restock a pharmacy's bulk medication supply?
    a. Mailing a hard copy of DEA Form 222 to the supplier
    b. Mailing a hard copy of DEA Form 224 to the supplier
    c. Faxing a copy of DEA Form 222 to the supplier
    d. Faxing a copy of DEA Form 224 to the supplier
    e. Sending an online order to the supplier with no additional form sent

81. Which of the following products is NOT required to be in tamper-evident packaging for retail sale?
    a. Acetaminophen tablets
    b. Children's diphenhydramine liquid
    c. Aspirin tablets
    d. Benzocaine/menthol lozenges
    e. Infant simethicone drops

82. A pharmacist may call a prescriber and receive verbal permission to change all of the following on a Schedule II prescription EXCEPT:
    a. Quantity
    b. Directions for use
    c. Drug name
    d. Drug strength
    e. Dosage form

83. A patient requests a copy of her prescription records from a community pharmacy. Within what time period must the pharmacy provide this information?
    a. 24 hours
    b. 3 days
    c. 7 days
    d. 10 days
    e. 30 days

84. Which of the following drugs has a REMS program due to a high frequency of birth defects?
    a. Lisinopril
    b. Thalidomide
    c. Zyprexa
    d. Atorvastatin
    e. Levothyroxine

85. Which law requires new drugs to be proven as safe and effective before approval?
    a. Poison Prevention Packaging Act
    b. Durham-Humphrey Amendment
    c. Kefauver-Harris Amendment
    d. Prescription Drug Marketing Act
    e. Drug Quality and Security Act

86. Anabolic steroids are classified under which controlled substance schedule under federal law?
    a. Schedule I
    b. Schedule II
    c. Schedule III
    d. Schedule IV
    e. Schedule V

87. Which act or amendment created the separation of drugs into two different categories, prescription (legend) and over-the-counter?
    a. Kefauver-Harris Amendment
    b. Omnibus Reconciliation Act
    c. Hatch-Waxman Amendment
    d. Durham-Humphrey Amendment
    e. Robinson-Patman Act

88. A patient picks up a prescription for Xarelto at a community pharmacy, but returns later in the day concerned that the prescription was filled with generic rivaroxaban. The pharmacist explains that the prescription was filled with the generic form of the medication because it was cheaper than using the brand name product. The patient asks if the generic will work as well as the brand name product. According to the pharmacist's drug reference, the two products have an FDA equivalency rating of AB. What is the proper interpretation of this code?
    a. The products are not bioequivalent, and the prescription should be filled only with brand name Xarelto
    b. The products have not been studied to determine bioequivalence, so a determination cannot be made
    c. The products have no known or suspected bioequivalence issues and are interchangeable
    d. The products may have actual or potential bioequivalence issues, but there is adequate evidence to use them interchangeably
    e. The code AB alone does not provide enough information to determine bioequivalence

89. DEA registration is NOT required for which of the following situations? Select ALL that apply.
    a. A nurse who is working in a physician's office where controlled substances are prescribed
    b. A pharmacist who regularly dispenses controlled substances at a community pharmacy
    c. A physician who occasionally prescribes controlled substances at a private clinic
    d. A patient who picks up a prescription for a newly prescribed controlled substance
    e. A pharmacy dispensing controlled substances

90. A drug manufacturer finds that bottles labeled "loratadine 10mg tablets" actually contain 5mg tablets, and issues a recall of the affected lot. Which of the following is true of this product?
    a. It is adulterated
    b. It is misbranded
    c. It is contaminated
    d. It is both adulterated and misbranded
    e. None of the above

91. A physician writes a prescription for ibuprofen 800mg tablets for a patient with rheumatoid arthritis. On the prescription, the physician adds a note that says, "please place this prescription and all future prescriptions in easy-open containers, as the patient is unable to open child-resistant bottles." Which of the following is true regarding this request?

    a. It is not valid because providers do not have the authority to request special packaging on a patient's behalf

    b. It is not valid because ibuprofen is not on the list of drugs exempt from the child-resistant packaging requirement under the Poison Prevention Packaging Act

    c. It is not valid because the provider must submit a separate signed form to make this request

    d. The ibuprofen can be dispensed in an easy-open container, but the blanket request to provide easy-open caps on all future prescriptions is not valid because only the patient can make such a request

    e. It is valid and a note should be made on the patient's profile to use easy-open containers on all prescriptions in the future

92. Which of the following would NOT be considered a potential part of a Risk Evaluation and Mitigation Strategy (REMS) program?

    a. Requiring special certification for pharmacies, practitioners, or health care settings that dispense a drug

    b. Requiring laboratory testing to ensure safe use of a drug

    c. Performing a financial assessment to ensure that a patient can afford a drug for the duration of treatment

    d. Providing a medication guide to patients which includes information about a drug

    e. Requiring that a patient enroll in a registry when they begin taking a drug

93. Retail containers of chewable low-dose 81mg aspirin (1.25 grain) must have special warnings for use in children including a warning regarding Reye's syndrome, and cannot contain more than:

    a. 10 tablets

    b. 30 tablets

    c. 36 tablets

    d. 48 tablets

    e. 60 tablets

94. Which of these is a valid DEA registration number for a mid-level practitioner?
    a. M11496023
    b. MT1200980
    c. CR5624112
    d. MM7411222
    e. BL115231

95. The FDA may require a medication guide be issued with certain prescriptions for which reason(s)? Select ALL that apply.
    a. When a drug has serious risks relative to benefits
    b. When patient adherence is crucial
    c. When the patient is a resident of a nursing home or other institution
    d. When drug information can prevent serious adverse effects
    e. When a pharmacist is unavailable to provide counseling on a new prescription

96. What act set the requirement that patients must be offered counseling on dispensed medications?
    a. OSHA 90
    b. DATA 90
    c. HCFA 90
    d. OPDP 90
    e. OBRA 90

97. Which of the following is/are NOT required to be packaged in a child-resistant container? Select ALL that apply.
    a. A container of 30 sublingual nitroglycerin tablets
    b. A methylprednisolone dose pack containing 21 tablets that are 4mg each
    c. A container of 100 aspirin tablets
    d. A prednisone dose pack containing 21 tablets that are 10mg each
    e. An albuterol inhaler

98. Prescription records must be kept for a minimum of _____ based on federal law.
    a. 1 year
    b. 2 years
    c. 3 years
    d. 4 years
    e. 5 years

99. A pharmacist dispenses a prescription for aripiprazole at an outpatient pharmacy. When is a medication guide required?
    a. Only for the first dispensing
    b. Every time the drug is filled, including refills
    c. Only if the patient requests
    d. The pharmacist may determine if a medication guide is necessary
    e. A medication guide is not required

100. To comply with Centers for Medicare and Medicaid Services (CMS) requirements, how often must a pharmacist conduct a drug regimen review for long-term care patients?
    a. At least once a week
    b. At least once a month
    c. At least once every 60 days
    d. At least once every 6 months
    e. Annually

Florida MPJE Practice Questions

1. Florida Board of Pharmacy members are appointed by the:
    a. Florida Pharmacists Association
    b. Senate
    c. DEA
    d. Governor
    e. Citizens

2. A practitioner that dispenses a Schedule III medication in the legal course of his/her practice in connection with a surgical procedure may not give more than a _____ day supply.
    a. Three
    b. Seven
    c. Ten
    d. Fourteen
    e. Thirty

3. The Florida Board of Pharmacy consists of:
    a. 11 members total
    b. 10 members total
    c. 9 members total
    d. 8 members total
    e. 7 members total

4. A bottle of metformin 1000 mg tablets has an expiration date of 10/23. What is the actual expiration date of the medication?
   a. 10/01/2023
   b. 10/15/2023
   c. 10/20/2023
   d. 10/31/2023
   e. None of the above

5. How many members on are the Drug Wholesale Distributor Advisory Council?
   a. Seven members
   b. Eight members
   c. Nine members
   d. Ten members
   e. Twelve members

6. How many pharmacists serve on the Florida Board of Pharmacy?
   a. 5 pharmacists
   b. 6 pharmacists
   c. 7 pharmacists
   d. 8 pharmacists
   e. 9 pharmacists

7. What constitutes an emergency oral prescription of a Schedule II controlled substance? Select ALL that apply.
   a. The patient has suffered severe trauma or a broken bone
   b. Immediate administration of the drug is necessary for proper treatment
   c. There is no alternative treatment available for the patient
   d. The patient did not receive a written prescription before leaving the prescriber's office
   e. The prescriber is not able to provide a written prescription at the time

8. Each pharmacy must have a continuous quality improvement (CQI) committee that meets once every:
   a. Week
   b. Two weeks
   c. Month
   d. Three months
   e. Year

9. A non-resident pharmacy mailing prescriptions to Florida residents must be open for a minimum of how many hours per week?
    a. Ten
    b. Twelve
    c. Twenty
    d. Thirty
    e. Forty

10. Which of the medications listed below are on Florida's negative drug formulary? Select ALL that apply.
    a. Abilify
    b. Crestor
    c. Lyrica
    d. Premarin
    e. Synthroid

11. How long can unclaimed prescriptions from a pharmacy be kept and reused for dispensing?
    a. Three months
    b. Six months
    c. One year
    d. Two years
    e. Only limit is the expiration date

12. How many witnesses must be present for the destruction of controlled substances at an institutional Class I pharmacy nursing home?
    a. One
    b. Two
    c. Three
    d. Four
    e. Five

13. Nurse practitioners may prescribe which of the following?
    a. Non-controlled substances
    b. Schedule III–V controlled substances
    c. Schedule II controlled substances
    d. Both (a) and (b)
    e. All of the above

14. A pharmacist should NOT dispense a generically equivalent drug product in which of the following cases? Select ALL that apply.
    a. The prescriber writes the words "MEDICALLY NECESSARY," in her or his own handwriting, on the face of a written prescription
    b. In the case of an oral prescription, the prescriber expressly indicates to the pharmacist that the brand name drug prescribed is medically necessary
    c. In the case of a prescription that is electronically generated and transmitted, the prescriber makes an overt act when transmitting the prescription to indicate that the brand name drug prescribed is medically necessary
    d. The brand name drug is less expensive than the generic equivalent
    e. The person presenting the prescription objects to a generic substitution

15. How many Board of Pharmacy members, at minimum, must be community pharmacists?
    a. Two
    b. Three
    c. Four
    d. Five
    e. Six

16. A pharmacy is destroying controlled substances which they can no longer use. A copy of the completed and witnessed Form DEA 41 must be mailed to the local DEA office no later than _____ after the destruction.
    a. 1 business day
    b. 3 business days
    c. 5 business days
    d. 7 days
    e. 14 days

17. The Board of Pharmacy grants a pharmacy permit for a pharmacy to open. However, the opening and operation of the pharmacy are going to be delayed. The permittee must notify the Board of Pharmacy within how many days of receiving the permit that the operation will be delayed?
    a. 7 days
    b. 14 days
    c. 15 days
    d. 30 days
    e. 60 days

18. At least one member serving on the Board of Pharmacy must be at least how old?
    a. 21 years
    b. 35 years
    c. 40 years
    d. 50 years
    e. 60 years

19. A backup copy of information from a pharmacy's data processing system must be kept and updated at least:
    a. Daily
    b. Weekly
    c. Monthly
    d. Quarterly
    e. Annually

20. Pharmacy interns must complete an immunization administration of at least _____ hours in order to become certified to immunize.
    a. 5 hours
    b. 10 hours
    c. 15 hours
    d. 20 hours
    e. 25 hours

21. How many hours of continuing education are pharmacists required to complete within two years prior to license renewal?
    a. 20 hours
    b. 30 hours
    c. 60 hours
    d. 90 hours
    e. 120 hours

22. A pharmacist from a pharmacy in Georgia calls requesting a prescription for Topamax to be transferred to their pharmacy. How should the pharmacist respond?
    a. Transfer the prescription after making sure it is a licensed pharmacist
    b. Tell the pharmacist only electronic transfers are permitted between states
    c. Say they will mail a copy of the prescription to the pharmacy
    d. Tell the pharmacist the prescription cannot be transferred outside the state
    e. Inform the pharmacist you must receive consent from the patient first

23. How many days must a pharmacist be allowed to produce documentation to address discrepancies found during a Medicaid audit?
    a. 5 days
    b. 7 days
    c. 10 days
    d. 15 days
    e. 30 days

24. The closest DEA field office must be notified within how many days before the proposed date of the transfer of pharmacy ownership?
    a. 3 days
    b. 7 days
    c. 14 days
    d. 30 days
    e. 60 days

25. Which controlled substances may be prescribed electronically through a system approved by the Board?
    a. Schedule V controlled substances
    b. Schedule IV–III controlled substances
    c. Schedule II controlled substances
    d. All of the above
    e. None of the above

26. As a general rule, without meeting specific criteria, a pharmacist may supervise up to _____ registered pharmacy technician(s) at one time.
    a. One
    b. Two
    c. Four
    d. Six
    e. Eight

27. The members of the Board of Pharmacy serve terms of:
    a. 2 years
    b. 4 years
    c. 5 years
    d. 6 years
    e. 8 years

28. What information must be documented in writing when Schedule III–V controlled substances are transferred to a new pharmacy? Select ALL that apply.
    a. Manufacturer name
    b. Dosage form
    c. Lot number
    d. Date transferred
    e. Pharmacy addresses

29. Modified Class II institutional pharmacies must establish a Pharmacy Services Committee that must meet at least once:
    a. Every month
    b. Every 3 months
    c. Every 6 months
    d. Annually
    e. Every 2 years

30. A customized medication package contains:
    a. 2 or more medications
    b. 3 or more medications
    c. 4 or more medications
    d. 5 or more medications
    e. 10 or more medications

31. How many hours of continuing education are pharmacy technicians required to complete every two years?
    a. 20 hours
    b. 30 hours
    c. 60 hours
    d. 90 hours
    e. 120 hours

32. How many continuing education hours for registered pharmacy technicians must be done through live presentation?
    a. Two hours
    b. Four hours
    c. Five hours
    d. Seven hours
    e. Ten hours

33. Dr. Hopkins calls in an emergency prescription of oxycodone for a patient. Within how many days must Dr. Hopkins provide a written prescription follow-up for the emergency order?
    a. 3 days
    b. 5 days
    c. 7 days
    d. 14 days
    e. A follow-up prescription does not need sent

34. Mr. Harold owned a pharmacy that just closed. Within how many days after closing must the pharmacy permit be returned?
    a. 3 days
    b. 7 days
    c. 10 days
    d. 14 days
    e. 30 days

35. How many continuing education hours for registered pharmacy technicians must be related to prevention of medication errors and pharmacy law every two years?
    a. Two hours
    b. Three hours
    c. Five hours
    d. Six hours
    e. Eight hours

36. A pharmacist can administer a long-acting antipsychotic medication at the direction of a physician if:

    I.   There is a protocol established with the physician

    II. There is a separate prescription for each injection

    III. The pharmacist completes a continuing education course

    a. I only
    b. II only
    c. I and II
    d. I and III
    e. I, II, and III

37. Original prescription file records must be kept for a minimum of how many years?
    a. 2 years
    b. 3 years
    c. 4 years
    d. 5 years
    e. 7 years

38. A pharmacy technician must have at least how many continuing education hours on the subject of HIV/AIDS upon the first license renewal?
    a. One hour
    b. Two hours
    c. Five hours
    d. Seven hours
    e. Ten hours

39. What is the maximum amount of a Schedule V substance of opium that can be sold to any one individual within a 48-hour period?
    a. 30 milligrams
    b. 60 milligrams
    c. 120 milligrams
    d. 240 milligrams
    e. 480 milligrams

40. A prescription filled at a central fill pharmacy must have which pharmacy or pharmacies identified on the prescription label?
    a. Central fill pharmacy by code
    b. Originating pharmacy by code
    c. Originating pharmacy by name and address
    d. Both (a) and (b)
    e. Both (a) and (c)

41. Who is authorized to be a witness of the destruction of controlled substances at an institutional Class I pharmacy nursing home (select ALL that apply)?
    a. Director of nursing
    b. Law enforcement officer
    c. Consultant pharmacist
    d. Medical assistant
    e. Social worker

42. Patient profiles at the pharmacy must contain all of the following EXCEPT:
    a. Gender
    b. Known drug interactions
    c. Chronic diseases
    d. Preferred drug brands
    e. Comprehensive list of relevant devices

43. Controlled substance medication containers must have a label bearing all of the following information EXCEPT:
    a. Name and address of the dispensing pharmacy
    b. Name of the prescriber and patient
    c. Directions for use of the prescribed substance
    d. Number of refills for the prescription
    e. Date of dispensing and prescription number

44. A prospective drug review consists of reviewing at least all of the following aspects EXCEPT:
    a. Reasonable dose
    b. Therapeutic duplication
    c. Incorrect duration of therapy
    d. Cost-effective alternatives
    e. Drug-drug interactions

45. A system in which all USP approved multi-dose units are physically connected is called a:
    a. Unit dose system
    b. Customized patient medication package
    c. Closed drug delivery system
    d. Restricted drug delivery system
    e. Packaged drug delivery system

46. Internet pharmacies must notify the Board of Pharmacy of a change in prescription department manager within how many days of the change?
    a. 7 days
    b. 10 days
    c. 15 days
    d. 30 days
    e. 45 days

47. Dr. Woodard is a pharmacist dispensing a Schedule II controlled substance to a patient. However, there is not enough of the medication to fill the entire prescription. Dr. Woodard dispenses a partial refill. Dr. Woodard must dispense the remaining amount within how long?
    a. 24 hours
    b. 48 hours
    c. 72 hours
    d. 7 days
    e. 14 days

48. For a consultant pharmacist that has the authority to order lab or clinical testing, they must have how many hours of continuing education related to lab and clinical testing?
    a. 1 hour
    b. 2 hours
    c. 3 hours
    d. 4 hours
    e. 5 hours

49. Non-resident pharmacies must report a change in the prescription department manager to the Florida Board of Pharmacy within how many days of the change?
    a. 10 days
    b. 14 days
    c. 15 days
    d. 30 days
    e. 45 days

50. Dr. Patel calls and explains he is calling in a Schedule II medication prescription due to an emergency situation. The pharmacist immediately reduces the order to writing on a prescription pad. The pharmacist can only dispense up to a _____ hour limit of medication in this situation.
    a. Twelve
    b. Twenty-four
    c. Thirty-six
    d. Forty-eight
    e. Seventy-two

51. At which type of institutional pharmacy are all medicinal drugs administered from individual prescription containers to the individual patient and in which medicinal drugs are not dispensed on the premises?
    a. Class I institutional pharmacy
    b. Modified Class I institutional pharmacy
    c. Class II institutional pharmacy
    d. Modified Class II institutional pharmacy
    e. Class III institutional pharmacy

52. What type of institutional pharmacy employs the services of a registered pharmacist or pharmacists who, in practicing institutional pharmacy, shall provide dispensing and consulting services on the premises to patients of that institution, for use on the premises of that institution?
    a. Class I institutional pharmacy
    b. Modified Class I institutional pharmacy
    c. Class II institutional pharmacy
    d. Modified Class II institutional pharmacy
    e. Class III institutional pharmacy

53. Mrs. Hartman comes to the pharmacy with the complaint of slightly painful urination. After talking with Mrs. Hartman more, the pharmacist decides it isn't necessary for her to schedule an appointment with a provider yet. The pharmacist can order and dispense phenazopyridine from the formulary for this patient, but it should be limited to a _____ day supply.
    a. Two
    b. Three
    c. Five
    d. Six
    e. Seven

54. A practitioner that dispenses a medication in the legal course of his/her practice in the manufacturer's package must dispense medications with a label that contains (select ALL that apply):
    a. Practitioner name
    b. Quantity of the medication
    c. Patient name
    d. Date of dispensing
    e. Number of authorized refills

55. A Modified Class II institutional pharmacy meets the requirements of a Class II institutional pharmacy, EXCEPT for these requirements:
    a. Space
    b. Personnel
    c. Equipment
    d. Both (a) and (b)
    e. Both (a) and (c)

56. A pharmacist must report to the law enforcement agency or sheriff any known or believed attempted fraudulent methods of obtaining a controlled substance either at the end of the next business day or within ___, whichever is later.
    a. 8 hours
    b. 12 hours
    c. 15 hours
    d. 24 hours
    e. 36 hours

57. Medicaid audits must be conducted by:
    a. A pharmacist licensed in Florida
    b. A physician licensed in Florida
    c. A nonresident pharmacist
    d. A financial officer from the Medicaid agency
    e. A member of the Florida Board of Pharmacy

58. An internet pharmacy must operate for a minimum of how many hours per week?
    a. 15 hours
    b. 20 hours
    c. 25 hours
    d. 30 hours
    e. 40 hours

59. Specialty pharmacies must notify the Board of Pharmacy of a change in responsible person within how many days of the change?
    a. 7 days
    b. 10 days
    c. 15 days
    d. 30 days
    e. 45 days

60. An institution allows any drug product to be stocked and/or prescribed without prior approval or review by the institution staff. What type of formulary does this institution have?
    a. Open formulary
    b. Closed formulary
    c. Restricted formulary
    d. Positive formulary
    e. Unrestricted formulary

61. The Florida Board of Pharmacy shall have at least how many public representatives serving on the Board?
    a. One
    b. Two
    c. Three
    d. Four
    e. None

62. A pharmacist who administered vaccinations must keep vaccine administration records for a minimum of how many years?
    a. 2 years
    b. 4 years
    c. 5 years
    d. 7 years
    e. 10 years

63. In order to enter into a protocol to allow a pharmacist to administer vaccines, what is the minimum amount a pharmacist must maintain for professional liability insurance?
    a. $50,000
    b. $100,000
    c. $150,000
    d. $200,000
    e. $300,000

64. A new substance that is not currently controlled may have "potential for abuse" if it has properties that create a substantial likelihood of being (select ALL that apply):
    a. Taken per the user's own initiative rather than based on how prescribed
    b. Used in amounts that are hazardous to user health or community safety

    c. Taken at the maximum prescribed PRN dose per day

    d. Used in amounts that cause the user to be slightly drowsy

    e. Diverted from legal use or distributed through illegal methods

65. All controlled substance prescriptions received for human patients must include (select ALL that apply):

    a. Date of issuance

    b. Number of refills

    c. Directions for use

    d. Address of prescriber

    e. Days supply

66. Up to how many hours of volunteer work every two years can a pharmacist receive continuing education hours serving the indigent or underserved population, or in areas of critical needs?

    a. Three

    b. Five

    c. Seven

    d. Ten

    e. Twelve

67. A pharmacy technician applicant wanting to become a technician through an apprenticeship must complete at least how many hours of a supervised apprenticeship by a Florida registered pharmacist?

    a. 250 hours

    b. 500 hours

    c. 1000 hours

    d. 1500 hours

    e. 2000 hours

68. When an audit of pharmacy records is conducted by a pharmacy benefits manager, the agency conducting the audit must give the pharmacy how much notice prior to the initial audit of the cycle?

    a. 3 days

    b. 5 days

    c. 7 days

    d. 15 days

    e. 30 days

69. Which type of prescriber may not administer or prescribe a Schedule II controlled substance?
    a. Optometrist
    b. Physician assistant
    c. Nurse practitioner
    d. Veterinarian
    e. Physician

70. What is the maximum supply of medications a prescriber at a Class II institution emergency department can dispense to a patient if the medication is necessary and community pharmacy services are not available or accessible?
    a. 12-hour supply
    b. 24-hour supply
    c. 36-hour supply
    d. 48-hour supply
    e. 72-hour supply

71. Dr. Robert Toms wrote a prescription for a Schedule II controlled substance and the pharmacist wants to verify the DEA number is legitimate. Which of the following is a valid DEA for Dr. Toms?
    a. PR1095834
    b. BT8410946
    c. FR1048570
    d. MT4882718
    e. AT3851424

72. Mrs. Sterling comes in with a prescription for Lyrica dated for today. What are the refill restrictions for this prescription?
    a. May not be refilled more than 1 time within a 2-month period
    b. May not be refilled more than 2 times within a 3-month period
    c. May not be refilled more than 4 times within a 6-month period
    d. May not be refilled more than 5 times within a 6-month period
    e. Can be refilled as often as prescribed within a 1-year period

73. A pharmacist must notify the Board of Pharmacy in writing within _____ days of the commencement of pharmacy practice in Florida after a pending disciplinary action.
    a. Seven

b. Ten

c. Fifteen

d. Twenty

e. Thirty

74. A prescription for dronabinol is called into the pharmacy. What is the maximum day supply a pharmacist can dispense for an oral Schedule III prescription?

    a. 7-day supply

    b. 14-day supply

    c. 30-day supply

    d. 60-day supply

    e. 90-day supply

75. When conducting a Medicaid audit, the agency conducting the audit must give the pharmacy how much notice prior to the initial audit of the cycle?

    a. 3 days

    b. 1 week

    c. 2 weeks

    d. 30 days

    e. 45 days

76. When a pharmacist is requesting information to receive a transferred prescription, they must record in writing or through electronic means (select ALL that apply):

    a. Prescription order and name of the drug

    b. Date of original dispensing and how much dispensed

    c. Number of remaining authorized refills

    d. Prescription number of the prescription on file

    e. Name of manufacturer of medication dispensed at original fill

77. Mr. Perry comes into the pharmacy on a Friday night and tells the pharmacist that he forgot to refill his prescription earlier and he just ran out of his Onfi. The pharmacist can dispense a one-time emergency refill of up to how many hours supply?

    a. Twenty-four

    b. Thirty-six

    c. Forty-eight

    d. Seventy-two

    e. Ninety-six

78. A pharmacy is damaged due to weather conditions and the pharmacy will have to be relocated to a new site while the old site is being rebuilt. The pharmacy owner must notify the Board of Pharmacy and local DEA office within how many hours of finding the pharmacy has been damaged?
   a. 12 hours
   b. 24 hours
   c. 48 hours
   d. 72 hours
   e. 96 hours

79. Nuclear pharmacies must notify the Board of Pharmacy of a change in responsible person within how many days of the change?
   a. 7 days
   b. 10 days
   c. 15 days
   d. 30 days
   e. 45 days

80. What is the maximum amount of a Schedule V substance of codeine that can be sold to any one individual within a 48-hour period?
   a. 30 milligrams
   b. 60 milligrams
   c. 120 milligrams
   d. 240 milligrams
   e. 480 milligrams

81. Which of the following meets the legal requirements for writing the drug quantity on a prescription for a controlled substance?
   a. 30
   b. 30 (thirty)
   c. Thirty (30)
   d. Both (a) and (b)
   e. Both (b) and (c)

82. The storage, compounding, dispensing, and Hot lab area of a nuclear pharmacy must be at least:
   a. 50 square feet
   b. 100 square feet

c. 150 square feet

d. 200 square feet

e. 250 square feet

83. An institutional pharmacy may only have medication samples upon written request from:
    a. The prescribing practitioner
    b. The pharmacy department manager
    c. The patient that will receive such samples
    d. Both (a) and (b)
    e. Both (a) and (c)

84. What is the first date of June in which an onsite audit of pharmacy records by a managed care company would be appropriate without consent from the pharmacy?
    a. June 2nd
    b. June 4th
    c. June 5th
    d. June 10th
    e. June 15th

85. Mr. Horn manages to make it to the pharmacy in the midst of a hurricane and requests a prescription refill on his blood pressure medication, but the pharmacist sees there are no refills left. The Governor had issued a state of emergency yesterday in the area due to the hurricane. What is the maximum day supply of the medication the pharmacy can dispense for an emergency fill?
    a. 3 days
    b. 7 days
    c. 14 days
    d. 30 days
    e. 45 days

86. Class II institutional pharmacy policy and procedures manuals must include a current list of (select ALL that apply):
    a. Pharmacist contract start dates
    b. Pharmacist names
    c. Pharmacist license numbers
    d. Pharmacist dates of birth
    e. Pharmacist addresses

87. Which date is the license renewal date for immunization certification licenses during the appropriate license renewal year?
    a. May 30th
    b. July 30th
    c. August 30th
    d. September 30th
    e. November 30th

88. How many hours of continuing education may be obtained in risk management through attending a full day or 8 hours of a disciplinary Board of Pharmacy meeting?
    a. Two hours
    b. Three hours
    c. Five hours
    d. Seven hours
    e. Eight hours

89. Along with providing the required information for a prescription transfer and recording "void" on the prescription record, the pharmacy with the original prescription must record on the prescription (select ALL that apply):
    a. Phone number of requesting pharmacy
    b. Name of requesting pharmacy
    c. Date of the transfer request
    d. Tax ID number of requesting pharmacy
    e. Name of requesting pharmacist

90. A pharmacy wants to destroy controlled substances that are not usable and knows that they must complete Form DEA-41. The destruction can be signed and witnessed by (Select ALL that apply):
    a. Consultant pharmacist of record and registered pharmacy technician
    b. Two D.E.A. agents
    c. Consultant pharmacist of record and a sworn law enforcement officer
    d. Florida Department of Health inspector and sworn law enforcement officer
    e. Prescription department manager and D.E.A. agent

91. Counterfeit-proof prescription pads must contain which of the following security features? Select ALL that apply.
    a. The pad must include a 3D security ribbon that is woven into the paper

b. The background color must be blue or green and resist reproduction

c. The pad or must be printed on artificial watermarked paper

d. The pad must resist erasures and alterations

e. The word "void" or "illegal" must appear on any photocopy

92. How many Board of Pharmacy members, at minimum, must be institutional pharmacists?

    a. No requirement

    b. One

    c. Two

    d. Three

    e. Four

93. A practitioner that dispenses medications in the legal course of his/her practice must dispense medications with a label that contains (select ALL that apply):

    a. Practitioner and patient name

    b. Number of authorized refills

    c. Quantity of the medication

    d. Date of dispensing

    e. Drug name, strength, and directions

94. What is the ratio of pharmacy interns to supervising pharmacists when an intern is administering vaccinations?

    a. 1 intern to 1 pharmacist

    b. 2 interns to 1 pharmacist

    c. 5 interns to 1 pharmacist

    d. 6 interns to 2 pharmacists

    e. Unlimited interns to 1 pharmacist

95. A nurse practitioner may not prescribe psychotropic drugs to patients under the age of:

    a. 5 years

    b. 7 years

    c. 13 years

    d. 16 years

    e. 18 years

96. A woman in her early twenties comes to the pharmacy with menstrual cramps and has no history of peptic ulcer disease. The pharmacist can order and dispense oral analgesics from the formulary for this patient, but it should be limited to a _____ day supply.
    a. Three
    b. Five
    c. Six
    d. Seven
    e. Ten

97. How many continuing education hours for pharmacists must be related to medication errors every two years prior to licensure expiration/renewal?
    a. Two hours
    b. Three hours
    c. Five hours
    d. Six hours
    e. Eight hours

98. What is the prescription drug monitoring program (PDMP) used in Florida?
    a. E-FORCE
    b. E-FLOR
    c. E-FORCSE
    d. E-FPDMP
    e. E-FCSE

99. How many continuing education hours for registered pharmacists must be done through live presentation, live video teleconference, or an interactive computer-based application?
    a. Two hours
    b. Four hours
    c. Five hours
    d. Seven hours
    e. Ten hours

100. A Class II institutional central fill pharmacy may deliver centrally filled medications to the:
    a. Patient
    b. Patient's caregiver

c. Originating pharmacy

d. Patient's healthcare provider

e. Both (a) and (c)

101. All pharmacists must complete _____ hours of continuing education on validating of prescriptions for controlled substances every two years before license renewal.

   a. Two

   b. Three

   c. Five

   d. Seven

   e. Ten

102. All of the following are able to prescribe therapeutic drugs in Florida within their scope of practice EXCEPT:

   a. Doctor of Psychology

   b. Doctor of Dental Medicine

   c. Physician Assistant

   d. Naturopath

   e. Doctor of Podiatric Medicine

103. What is the maximum amount of a Schedule V substance of dihydrocodeine that can be sold to any one individual within a 48-hour period?

   a. 30 milligrams

   b. 60 milligrams

   c. 120 milligrams

   d. 240 milligrams

   e. 480 milligrams

104. A pharmacist has been retired for 6 years and has decided he wants to start practicing pharmacy again. What must this pharmacist do in order to apply for an active license in the state of Florida?

   a. Complete 60 hours of continuing education within 2 years of applying

   b. Take and pass the jurisprudence exam and the NAPLEX

   c. Attend a live Florida law review equivalent to 5 hours of continuing education

   d. Take and pass the jurisprudence exam only

   e. Take and pass an appropriate therapeutics test administered by the state

105. How many hours of a continuing education course must a pharmacist receive regarding safe and effective administration of behavioral health and antipsychotic injections to be able to administer long-acting antipsychotics?
    a. 2 hours
    b. 4 hours
    c. 5 hours
    d. 8 hours
    e. 10 hours

106. The pharmacist manager should make how many backup tapes/disks of drug inventory and prescription information if the pharmacy will be closed or evacuated due to a hurricane or other national emergency?
    a. One
    b. Two
    c. Three
    d. Four
    e. None

107. Inventory of controlled substances must be completed at least once every:
    a. 3 months
    b. 6 months
    c. 1 year
    d. 2 years
    e. 3 years

108. What is the days supply limit for dispensing a Schedule II opioid for acute pain, unless otherwise determined medically necessary by a prescriber?
    a. Two days
    b. Three days
    c. Five days
    d. Seven days
    e. Fourteen days

109. Unless the amount or day limit is otherwise specified, a pharmacist registered as a dispensing practitioner can prescribe and dispense approved medications for up to a _____ day supply.
    a. Seven
    b. Fourteen

c. Twenty-one
d. Thirty
e. Thirty-four

110. An internet pharmacy must operate for a minimum of how many days per week?
    a. 3 days
    b. 4 days
    c. 5 days
    d. 6 days
    e. 7 days

111. What formulary is composed of medicinal drugs that demonstrate clinically significant biological or therapeutic inequivalence and potential adverse effects or threats if substituted?
    a. Positive formulary
    b. Inequivalence formulary
    c. Non-interchangeable formulary
    d. Negative formulary
    e. Non-substitution formulary

112. A prescriber who calls in an emergency oral Schedule II controlled substance prescription must deliver the original written prescription to the pharmacy within how many days after authorizing the oral prescription?
    a. One day
    b. Two days
    c. Three days
    d. Five days
    e. Seven days

113. On the day of a pharmacy closing, the permittee of the pharmacy must (select ALL that apply):
    a. Deliver prescription files to a different pharmacy that is close in proximity
    b. Notify the Board of Pharmacy in writing of the pharmacy closure
    c. Fix a sign to the front entrance advising the public of the pharmacy where prescription files were transferred
    d. Advise the Board of Pharmacy of which pharmacy received the prescription files
    e. Return the pharmacy permit to the Board of Pharmacy

114. Pharmacists who are on the Board of Pharmacy must have been engaged in pharmacy practice in Florida for at least _____ year(s) before appointment to the Board.
    a. One
    b. Two
    c. Three
    d. Four
    e. Five

115. What is the name of the Florida online immunization registry that helps keep immunization records?
    a. Florida VAX
    b. Florida ImpactSIIS
    c. Florida SHOTS
    d. Florida VACC
    e. None of the above

116. How often must a community pharmacy with a compounding room be inspected if it has passed inspections for the previous most current three years with no disciplinary actions?
    a. Twice a year
    b. Once a year
    c. Every two years
    d. Every three years
    e. Every five years

117. Dr. Mentch is a pharmacist with a nuclear pharmacist license that has been practicing in another state and is now going to be practicing in Florida. He has not completed the didactic and experiential training requirements for nuclear pharmacists in the past 7 years. How many hours must Dr. Mentch have practiced nuclear pharmacy in the past 7 years in order to practice in Florida without the training requirements?
    a. 500 hours
    b. 750 hours
    c. 1000 hours
    d. 1080 hours
    e. 2050 hours

118. A terminally ill patient from a Long Term Care Facility (LTCF) wants their Schedule II controlled substance dispensed as a partial prescription. How should the pharmacist respond?
    a. Fill the whole prescription–partial dispensing is not allowed unless the pharmacist is unable to fill the entire quantity for Schedule II substances
    b. Fill the whole prescription–partial dispensing for Schedule II substances is not allowed under any circumstances
    c. Partially dispense the prescription–partial dispensing of Schedule II substances may be done for terminally ill LTCF patients
    d. Partially dispense the prescription–partial dispensing of Schedule II substances is allowed for anyone under any circumstances
    e. Verify with the prescriber it is acceptable to partially dispense the prescription before doing so

119. A pharmacist that suspects a prescriber is involved in controlled substance diversion should report the prescriber to the:
    a. Medical Board
    b. Board of Pharmacy
    c. Department of Professional Affairs
    d. Board of Medical Practice
    e. Department of Health

120. A pharmacist engaged in sterile compounding may supervise up to _____ registered pharmacy technicians at one time with Board approval.
    a. Two
    b. Three
    c. Four
    d. Six
    e. Eight

121. How often must a community pharmacy with a compounding room be inspected if it is the first year of operation?
    a. Twice a year
    b. Once a year
    c. Every two years
    d. Every three years
    e. Every five years

122. At a pharmacy where drugs are not dispensed and there is no sterile compounding, a pharmacist may supervise up to _____ registered pharmacy technicians at one time with Board approval.
    a. Three
    b. Five
    c. Six
    d. Eight
    e. Ten

123. A non-resident pharmacy must be available through a toll-free telephone number for a minimum of how many hours per week?
    a. Ten
    b. Twelve
    c. Twenty
    d. Thirty
    e. Forty

124. What is the first date of November in which an onsite Medicaid audit would be appropriate?
    a. November 2nd
    b. November 3rd
    c. November 6th
    d. November 10th
    e. November 14th

125. A local nursing home is repackaging medications from patients' prescription bottles into unit dose containers. Which of the following is true?
    a. The medications are considered misbranded
    b. The medications are considered adulterated
    c. The medication expiration date changes to 3 months from the repackaging date
    d. The medication expiration date changes to 1 month from the repackaging date
    e. There is no problem with the nursing home repackaging the medications

126. Applicants for a consultant pharmacist license must successfully complete a consultant pharmacist course of at least how many hours?
    a. Five

b. Eight

c. Twelve

d. Fifteen

e. Twenty

127. Who must notify the Board of Pharmacy when there is a theft or significant loss of any controlled substance?

    a. Any pharmacist

    b. Pharmacy department manager

    c. Any pharmacy technician

    d. Both (a) and (b)

    e. All of the above

128. Within how many days of discovering theft or loss of a controlled substance must the Board of Pharmacy be notified?

    a. One day

    b. Two days

    c. Three days

    d. Five days

    e. Seven days

129. Controlled drugs stocked within a Type "A" Modified Class II Institutional Pharmacy must be stocked in unit size not to exceed _____.

    a. 20 dosage units

    b. 50 dosage units

    c. 100 dosage units

    d. 250 dosage units

    e. 500 dosage units

130. Mr. Newman is a pharmacist that is going on his lunch break. He is the only pharmacist working in the store that day. His meal must not be more than how many minutes?

    a. 10 minutes

    b. 15 minutes

    c. 20 minutes

    d. 30 minutes

    e. 45 minutes

131. Class II institutional pharmacy remote medication order processing records identifying the person who processed the orders must be readily retrievable for at least:
    a. One year
    b. Two years
    c. Three years
    d. Four years
    e. Five years

132. Who may have the keys and/or means to access the prescription department of a pharmacy?
    a. Pharmacist
    b. Pharmacy intern
    c. Pharmacy technician
    d. Both (a) and (b)
    e. Both (a) and (c)

133. A prescription copy may be issued to:
    a. A pharmacist at another retail pharmacy
    b. The patient or patient's caregiver
    c. The patient's prescriber
    d. Both (a) and (c)
    e. Both (b) and (c)

134. Pharmacies must back up data from their data processing system at least every:
    a. One day
    b. Three days
    c. Seven days
    d. Fourteen days
    e. Thirty days

135. Which of the following are true of written prescriptions for medicinal drugs? Select ALL that apply.
    a. Must be typed
    b. Must contain the name of the prescribing practitioner
    c. Must contain the name and strength of the drug, and the quantity prescribed
    d. Must contain the directions for use of the drug
    e. Must be signed by the prescribing practitioner on the day when issued

136. What is the supervision limit for interns who are foreign pharmacy graduates?
    a. One pharmacist to one intern
    b. One pharmacist to two interns
    c. One pharmacist to three interns
    d. One pharmacist to four interns
    e. A pharmacist may supervise any number of foreign graduate interns

137. The period of time covered by a Medicaid audit may not exceed _____.
    a. Six months
    b. One year
    c. Two years
    d. Three years
    e. Five years

138. The following are Modified Class II institutional pharmacies (select ALL that apply):
    a. Alcoholism treatment center
    b. Rapid in/out surgical center
    c. Hospital pharmacy
    d. Community retail pharmacy
    e. Correctional institution

139. All of the following can be provided in an emergency refill EXCEPT:
    a. A one-time emergency refill of a 72-hour supply of prescribed medication
    b. A one-time emergency refill of one vial of insulin to treat diabetes
    c. A one-time emergency refill of up to a 72-hour supply of a Schedule V medication
    d. A 30-day supply of medication for a chronic condition in an area where the Governor issued an emergency order
    e. A 30-day supply of a Schedule II drug in an area under an emergency order

140. A consultant pharmacist must provide on-site consultations at Modified Class II institutional pharmacies at least:
    a. Once a week
    b. Twice a month
    c. Once a month
    d. Once every 2 months
    e. Once every 3 months

141. Which date is the license renewal date for community pharmacists during the appropriate license renewal year?
    a. June 30th
    b. July 30th
    c. August 30th
    d. September 30th
    e. October 30th

142. A prescription department manager is allowed to be the manager at how many pharmacies?
    a. One
    b. Two
    c. Three
    d. Four
    e. Five

143. Which of the following are Schedule IV medications? Select ALL that apply.
    a. Alprazolam
    b. Eszopiclone
    c. Lorazepam
    d. Testosterone
    e. Zaleplon

144. Hard-copy printouts of prescription data must contain all of the following prescription information EXCEPT:
    a. Prescriber name
    b. Quantity dispensed
    c. Initials or identification code of dispensing pharmacist
    d. Number of refills remaining
    e. Drug strength

145. How often must a community pharmacy with a compounding room be inspected if it has failed inspections during the first two years or was disciplined?
    a. Twice a year
    b. Once a year
    c. Every two years
    d. Every three years
    e. Every five years

146. The controlled substances "Caution" warning statement must be on the label of which controlled substances in Florida?
    a. Schedule V controlled substances
    b. Schedule III– IV controlled substances
    c. Schedule II controlled substances
    d. Both (b) and (c)
    e. All of the above

147. Which date is the pharmacy permit renewal for the appropriate renewal year?
    a. January 28th
    b. February 28th
    c. April 28th
    d. June 28th
    e. September 28th

148. How often are pharmacy permits renewed?
    a. Every six months
    b. Every nine months
    c. Every one year
    d. Every two years
    e. Every three years

149. In order to obtain a license as a nuclear pharmacist, a pharmacist must complete _____ hours of didactic instruction and supervised practical experience in nuclear pharmacy.
    a. 1000 hours
    b. 800 hours
    c. 500 hours
    d. 300 hours
    e. 200 hours

150. What is the system called when the control of customized patient medication packages or unit doses are maintained by the facility and not the patient?
    a. Unit dose system
    b. Open drug delivery system
    c. Closed drug delivery system
    d. Restricted drug delivery system
    e. Packaged drug delivery system

151. The drug formulary at a Type "A" Modified Class II institutional pharmacy cannot have more than how many medicinal drugs?
    a. Ten
    b. Fifteen
    c. Thirty
    d. Forty-five
    e. Sixty

152. A terminally ill LTCF patient has a prescription for a Schedule II controlled substance. The prescription may be partially dispensed for up to:
    a. 72 hours
    b. 30 days after the first fill
    c. 30 days from the prescription issuance
    d. 60 days after the first fill
    e. 60 days from the prescription issuance

153. A pharmacist not engaged in sterile compounding may supervise up to _____ registered pharmacy technicians at one time with Board approval.
    a. Two
    b. Three
    c. Four
    d. Six
    e. Eight

154. If a community pharmacy is confirming records of dispensing by a daily hard-copy printout, the printout needs produced within _____ of the date on which the dispensing took place.
    a. Twenty-four hours
    b. Forty-eight hours
    c. Seventy-two hours
    d. Five days
    e. Seven days

155. Prescriptions for Schedule II controlled substances can be faxed when they are for (select ALL that apply):
    a. Compounding for direct administration to a patient
    b. An inpatient about to be discharged to pick up from an outpatient pharmacy
    c. Patients residing in a long-term care facility

d. Patients residing in hospice care certified by Medicare

e. Ambulatory patients that were discharged with a broken bone

156. Each pharmacist that dispensed or refilled medications on the date of dispensing must sign the daily hard-copy printout of prescription records within how many days of the dispensing date?

  a. Two days

  b. Three days

  c. Five days

  d. Seven days

  e. Fourteen days

157. Instead of using a daily hard-copy printout, a pharmacy can maintain a signature log book of each pharmacist that is using the data processing system. When does the log book need signed by each pharmacist for the particular date they were dispensing?

  a. The day of dispensing

  b. Within two days

  c. Within three days

  d. Within five days

  e. Within seven days

158. Medication labels from unit dose systems must contain all of the following EXCEPT:

  a. Patient name

  b. Prescriber name

  c. Prescription number

  d. Directions for use

  e. Fill date

159. A nuclear pharmacist must complete an additional _____ hours of approved coursework that relates to nuclear pharmacy every two years.

  a. Four

  b. Ten

  c. Fifteen

  d. Twenty-four

  e. Thirty

160. A pharmacist must have at least how many hours of continuing education on the subject of HIV/AIDS upon the first license renewal?
   a. One hour
   b. Two hours
   c. Five hours
   d. Seven hours
   e. Ten hours

161. An extended days supply of a Schedule II opioid for acute pain is deemed medically necessary by the prescriber. Since deemed medically necessary by the prescriber, rather than the 3 days supply limit, it can be extended to a limit of:
   a. Two days
   b. Three days
   c. Five days
   d. Seven days
   e. Fourteen days

162. Which prescriptions must include a written and numerical notation of the quantity prescribed (select ALL that apply)?
   a. Non-controlled medications
   b. Schedule II controlled substance prescriptions
   c. Schedule III controlled substance prescriptions
   d. Schedule IV controlled substance prescriptions
   e. Schedule V controlled substance prescriptions

163. Which date is the license renewal date for consultant pharmacists during the appropriate license renewal year?
   a. January 31st
   b. April 31st
   c. September 31st
   d. October 31st
   e. December 31st

164. A pharmacist must complete at least _____ hours of supervised practical experience in nuclear pharmacy, along with didactic training requirements, to become a certified nuclear pharmacist.
   a. 600
   b. 500

c. 300

d. 200

e. 100

165. Labels on compounded drugs provided for office use must include (Select ALL that apply):

    a. The name, address, and phone number of the compounding pharmacy

    b. The name and strength of the preparation

    c. The pharmacy's lot number

    d. The date the drug was compounded and the pharmacist's name

    e. The quantity or amount in the container

166. Members of the Drug Wholesale Advisory Council serve a term of how many years?

    a. Two years

    b. Four years

    c. Five years

    d. Six years

    e. Eight years

167. A chain pharmacy wants to centralize certain controlled substance records in a single location. The pharmacy must notify the DEA how many days before doing so, and in what form must the notification be?

    a. 7 days; computerized

    b. 7 days; writing

    c. 14 days; computerized

    d. 14 days; writing

    e. 30 days; writing

168. How many hours of a continuing education course in vaccine administration must a pharmacist complete in order to be able to become licensed to administer vaccinations?

    a. 5 hours

    b. 10 hours

    c. 15 hours

    d. 20 hours

    e. 25 hours

169. Log book records of dispensing pharmacist signatures verifying the prescription records must be kept for a period of _____ from the date of dispensing.
   a. Six months
   b. One year
   c. Two years
   d. Three years
   e. Four years

170. A log of the sale of Schedule V OTC products must be kept for a period of at least:
   a. 6 months
   b. 9 months
   c. 1 year
   d. 2 years
   e. 5 years

171. In which type of institutional pharmacy are all medicinal drugs administered from individual prescription containers to the individual patient?
   a. Class I
   b. Class II
   c. Class III
   d. Modified Class I
   e. Modified Class II

172. Oral prescriptions for controlled substances must be reduced to writing:
   a. Immediately
   b. Within 30 minutes
   c. Within 1 hour
   d. Within 2 hours
   e. Within the business day

173. A practitioner that dispenses controlled substance medications in the legal course of his/her practice must dispense medications with a label that contains (select ALL that apply):
   a. Practitioner and patient name
   b. Number of authorized refills
   c. Quantity of the medication
   d. Prescription number
   e. Directions for use

174. A Medicaid audit report must be delivered to the pharmacist within _____ days after the conclusion of the audit.
    a. Fifteen
    b. Thirty
    c. Forty-five
    d. Sixty
    e. Ninety

175. Who must notify the Board of a change in the prescription department manager at a community pharmacy?
    a. Pharmacy owner
    b. New prescription department manager
    c. Old prescription department manager
    d. Both (a) and (b)
    e. Both (a) and (c)

176. Controlled substance prescriptions may be written with (select ALL that apply):
    a. A typewriter
    b. A pen
    c. A number 2 pencil
    d. A computer and then printed out
    e. An indelible pencil

177. Dispensing of controlled substances must be reported through a prescription drug monitoring program (PDMP):
    a. By the end of the next business day after dispensing
    b. Within 48 hours of dispensing
    c. Within 72 hours of dispensing
    d. Within 5 days of dispensing
    e. Within 7 days of dispensing

178. Loss of information from a data processing system in a pharmacy must be reported to the Board of Pharmacy within how many days of discovering the loss?
    a. 3 days
    b. 5 days
    c. 7 days
    d. 10 days
    e. 15 days

179. A pharmacist did not have enough medication to fill a hydrocodone prescription, so the pharmacist partially dispensed it, using the quantity on hand. The pharmacist must record on the prescription (select ALL that apply):
    a. That it was partially filled
    b. Reason for partially dispensing
    c. Partial quantity dispensed
    d. Date of dispensing the partial quantity
    e. The date the rest needs dispensed by

180. Non-resident pharmacies must report a change in location to the Florida Board of Pharmacy within how many days of the change?
    a. 10 days
    b. 14 days
    c. 15 days
    d. 30 days
    e. 45 days

181. The following are included on the negative formulary (select ALL that apply):
    a. Digitoxin
    b. Conjugated estrogen
    c. Testosterone
    d. Dicumarol
    e. Aminophylline

182. The label affixed to the immediate inner container of a radiopharmaceutical to be distributed must include all of the following EXCEPT:
    a. The standard radiation symbol
    b. The chemical form
    c. The words "Caution Radioactive Material"
    d. The prescription order number of the radiopharmaceutical
    e. The name of the patient or the words "Physician's Use Only."

183. Which type of pharmacy or pharmacies may store drugs in bulk?
    a. Modified Class II Type A pharmacies
    b. Modified Class II Type B pharmacies
    c. Modified Class II Type C pharmacies
    d. Both (a) and (b)
    e. Both (b) and (c)

184. Certified optometrists must complete a 20-hour board-approved course in order to prescribe which of the following?
    a. Topical ocular pharmaceutical agents
    b. Oral ocular pharmaceutical agents
    c. Antidiabetic medications
    d. Antihypertensive medications
    e. None of the above

185. At what age can a person start purchasing pseudoephedrine-containing products in the state of Florida?
    a. 13 years
    b. 16 years
    c. 18 years
    d. 21 years
    e. 25 years

186. When ownership of medications is being transferred to a new owner, who must be notified, and who must they be notified by?
    a. Board of Pharmacy; transferee pharmacy
    b. Department of Health; transferee pharmacy
    c. Board of Pharmacy; transferor pharmacy
    d. Department of Health; transferor pharmacy
    e. Public Health Department; transferor pharmacy

187. How often must a nursing home consultant pharmacist review documents of controlled substance destruction?
    a. Once a week
    b. Once a month
    c. Once every 3 months
    d. Once every 6 months
    e. Once a year

188. A nurse practitioner may prescribe Schedule II controlled substances for up to a:
    a. 3-day supply
    b. 7-day supply
    c. 10-day supply
    d. 14-day supply
    e. 30-day supply

189. How many hours of continuing education for safe and effective vaccine administration must a certified pharmacist immunizer complete every 2 years before their license renewal?
   a. 1 hour
   b. 2 hours
   c. 3 hours
   d. 4 hours
   e. 5 hours

190. A pharmacy must be open a minimum of how many hours per week?
   a. 15 hours
   b. 20 hours
   c. 25 hours
   d. 30 hours
   e. 40 hours

191. The prescription drug monitoring program (PDMP) must be consulted each time a controlled substance prescription is dispensed for individuals:
   a. 7 and older
   b. 13 and older
   c. 16 and older
   d. 18 and older
   e. 21 and older

192. Under what circumstances may a Florida pharmacy sell or dispense expired medications to the public?
   a. Within 3 days after the expiration date
   b. Within 7 days after the expiration date
   c. Within 1 month after the expiration date
   d. Only during a state of emergency
   e. Expired medications may never be sold to the public

193. What is true of counterfeit-resistant prescription pads? Select ALL that apply.
   a. Veterinarians must use them when writing controlled substance prescriptions
   b. They may only be purchased from approved vendors
   c. Practitioners are required to have their license number pre-printed on them
   d. MDs must use them for all written prescriptions
   e. MDs must use them for all written controlled substance prescriptions

194. Upon the request from a law enforcement officer, a hard copy printout of controlled substances dispensed must be produced within:
    a. 12 hours
    b. 24 hours
    c. 36 hours
    d. 48 hours
    e. 72 hours

195. Hard copy printouts of controlled substances dispensed that are printed for law enforcement officers must cover a period of at least how many days of dispensing?
    a. 7 days
    b. 14 days
    c. 30 days
    d. 60 days
    e. 90 days

196. Information required to be on an issued prescription form includes all of the following EXCEPT:
    a. Patient phone number
    b. Prescriber profession/credentials
    c. Patient date of birth or age
    d. Prescriber address
    e. Medication dosage form

197. Summarization records from each pharmacy's continuous quality improvement (CQI) committee must be kept for a period of at least:
    a. 1 year
    b. 2 years
    c. 3 years
    d. 4 years
    e. 5 years

198. Community pharmacy inspections are done by persons from:
    a. The Department of Health
    b. The Board of Pharmacy
    c. The Drug Enforcement Administration
    d. Centers for Medicaid and Medicare
    e. Both (a) and (b)

199. Redistribution (transfer) of controlled substances to a practitioner must not exceed _____ percent of the total number of all controlled substances dispensed by the pharmacy during the 12-month DEA registration period.
    a. Three
    b. Five
    c. Seven
    d. Ten
    e. Fifteen

200. A non-resident pharmacy sending prescriptions to Florida residents must disclose the location, names, and titles of all pharmacists dispensing medications to Florida residents at least:
    a. Every month
    b. Every 3 months
    c. Every 6 months
    d. Every year
    e. Every 2 years

Answer Index — Federal Questions

1 – a

The Food, Drug, and Cosmetic Act (FDCA) requires all new drugs to be proven safe for their labeled use before they can be marketed to patients. This act was passed in 1938 after a drug called elixir sulfanilamide caused mass poisonings and over a hundred deaths in the United States.

2 – a

Drug recalls are classified as Class I, II, or III, from most severe to least severe. A Class I recall is when a product may cause serious adverse health issues or death. A Class II recall is when a product has a low likelihood of causing serious adverse effects, but may cause some temporary or reversible adverse effects. A Class III recall is when a product is not likely to cause adverse health consequences.

3 – d

The Drug Enforcement Administration (DEA) is part of the U.S. Department of Justice and is responsible for the federal CSA. The Controlled Substances Act is available online on the DEA website. HIPAA is usually enforced by the Department of Health and Human Services.

4 – d

The Orange Book (the official title is "Approved Drug Products with Therapeutic Equivalence Evaluations") is the primary source for determining the therapeutic equivalency of drugs. The Purple Book lists biological products that are considered biosimilars and provides interchangeability evaluations for these products. The Red Book contains drug pricing information. The Green Book is for FDA-approved animal drugs.

5 – d

No directions for administration are necessary for oral drug products. However, if drugs are not for oral use, then the specific route(s) of administration must be stated.

Label requirements for the manufacturer container include: name and address of the manufacturer/packer/distributor, name of drug or product, net quantity packaged, weights of each active ingredient, route(s) of administration for non-oral medications, manufacturer control or lot number, expiration date, special storage instructions if applicable, and the federal legend (e.g. "Rx only").

6 – b

According to the DEA Pharmacist's Manual, a controlled substance listed in schedules II, III, IV, or V which is not a prescription drug as determined under the Federal Food, Drug, and Cosmetic Act may be dispensed by a pharmacist to a purchaser at retail, provided that:

- The dispensing is made only by a pharmacist and not by a non-pharmacist employee even if under the supervision of a pharmacist (although after the pharmacist has fulfilled his or her professional and legal responsibilities, the actual cash transaction, credit transaction, or delivery may be completed by a non-pharmacist)

- Not more than 240 cc. (8 ounces) of any such controlled substance containing opium, nor more than 120 cc. (4 ounces) of any other such controlled substance, nor more than 48 dosage units of any such controlled substance containing opium, nor more than 24 dosage units of any other such controlled substance, may be dispensed at retail to the same purchaser in any given 48-hour period

- The purchaser is at least 18 years of age

- The pharmacist requires every purchaser of a controlled substance not known to him to furnish suitable identification (including proof of age where appropriate)

- A bound record book is maintained by the pharmacist which contains the name and address of the purchaser, the name and quantity of the controlled substance purchased, the date of each purchase, and the name or initials of the pharmacist who dispensed the substance to the purchaser

- A prescription is not required for distribution or dispensing of the substance pursuant to any other federal, state or local law

- Central fill pharmacies may not dispense controlled substances at the retail level to a purchaser.

7 – a

A DEA Form 106, titled "Report of Theft or Loss of Controlled Substances," is a form that must be filled out and submitted to the DEA upon discovery of theft or significant loss of controlled substances. There is a section of the DEA Form 106 that allows the user to list out the controlled substances and quantities that were stolen or lost. Submitting a DEA Form 106 formally documents the situation and the pharmacy should retain a copy for their records. The DEA must also immediately be contacted by phone, fax, or brief written message to alert them of the situation. The local authorities should also be alerted.

There is no DEA Form 108. DEA Form 222 is for ordering Schedule II controlled substances. DEA Form 224 is for registration with the DEA. DEA Form 363 is for narcotic treatment facilities.

8 – d

Pentobarbital is a Schedule II controlled substance. It is a barbiturate. Schedule II controlled substances include but are not limited to: opiates and opioids, amphetamines and dextroamphetamine salts, pentobarbital, secobarbital, and phencyclidine. Mescaline is a Schedule I controlled substance. Butabarbital is a Schedule III controlled substance. Modafinil is a Schedule IV controlled substance. Finally, buprenorphine is a Schedule III controlled substance.

9 – c

A non-preserved aqueous oral formulation made from commercially available drug products has a maximum beyond-use date (BUD) of 14 days when refrigerated. Preserved aqueous formulations, such as topical and mucosal liquids or semisolid preparations, may have a BUD of up to 35 days, while non-aqueous dosage forms like capsules or powders have a BUD of up to 180 days.

The BUD must not exceed the expiration date of any ingredient used, and formulations with unstable components may require shorter BUDs.

10 – c

Here is a summary of DEA forms to know:

- DEA Form 222 is for ordering Schedule I or II controlled substances

- DEA Form 224 is for registering a new pharmacy

- DEA Form 363 is for new registration applications for narcotic treatment programs

- DEA Form 106 is for reporting loss

- DEA Form 41 is for drug destruction.

11 – c

The Food and Drug Administration has developed four distinct approaches to making certain types of new drugs available as rapidly as possible. The four approaches are:

- Fast track

- Breakthrough therapy

- Accelerated approval

- Priority review

Fast track is an expedited review process intended for drugs that treat serious conditions and fill an unmet medical need. Breakthrough therapy is a process designed to expedite the development and review of drugs which may demonstrate substantial improvement over available therapy. Accelerated approval is for drugs with long-term endpoints that are hard to measure during clinical trials, such as a decrease in mortality or increase in survival. These drugs are approved based on a surrogate endpoint. Finally, the priority review designation means the FDA's goal is to take action on the application within six months. "Instant approval" is not an FDA process.

12 - d

Schedule II controlled substances can be transferred in all of the given scenarios except for a researcher transferring Schedule II controlled substances to a pharmacy to be dispensed to patients. Researchers must be authorized to conduct research with Schedule II controlled substances. Researchers may transfer Schedule II controlled substances to another authorized researcher for the purpose of research. Researchers may not transfer Schedule II controlled substances to a pharmacy.

13 – b

Once a pharmacy has filled and dispensed a medication, the prescription is legally owned by the pharmacy and the original prescription can't be returned to the patient. However, it is acceptable to make a copy for the patient or the prescriber if needed. The prescription can be transferred to another pharmacy (if legal depending on the schedule and number of refills remaining), but the pharmacy that originally filled the prescription must retain the original copy.

14 - b

When purchasing Schedule II controlled substances, the pharmacy (purchaser) will fill out a DEA Form 222 and submit it to the supplier. The supplier receives the original form. The purchaser is required to make a copy of the original DEA Form 222 for their records. This copy can be retained in paper or electronic form. The purchaser does not have the option of keeping the original form.

15 – b

A Class II drug recall occurs when the product may cause temporary or medically reversible adverse effects, but the probability of serious adverse effects is remote.

16 – c

National Drug Codes (NDCs) are drug identification numbers that are unique to each drug manufactured. The NDC contains 3 sets of numbers:

1) The first set is either a 4- or 5-digit number and represents the manufacturer.

2) The second set is a 4-digit number that represents the identity of the drug.

3) The third set is a 2-digit number that is the product package size, such as the bottle count, blister packs, etc.

For example, we might have levothyroxine 50 mcg that is supplied as a 100-count bottle and a 500-count bottle from the same manufacturer. The NDC code will be the same except for the last 2 numbers because the bottle count sizes are different.

17 – e

Good Manufacturing Practice (GMP) is a set of regulations that determines minimum standards for pharmaceutical manufacturing in the U.S. The purpose of GMP is to uphold the safety and quality of drug products.

18 – b

According to the DEA Pharmacist's Manual, these are the criteria for an individual practitioner issuing multiple prescriptions for up to a 90-day supply of a Schedule II controlled substance:

- Each separate prescription is issued for a legitimate medical purpose by an individual practitioner acting in the usual course of professional practice

- The individual practitioner provides written instructions on each prescription (other than the first prescription, if the prescribing practitioner intends for that prescription to be filled immediately) indicating the earliest <u>date</u> on which a pharmacy may fill each prescription

- The individual practitioner concludes that providing the patient with multiple prescriptions in this manner does not create an undue risk of diversion or abuse

- The issuance of multiple prescriptions is permissible under the applicable state laws

- The individual practitioner complies fully with all other applicable federal requirements as well as any additional requirements under state law.

19 – d

Based on federal law, Schedule III and IV controlled substances can be refilled up to 5 times in a 6-month period from the date the prescription was written. Some states also apply this refill rule to Schedule V controlled substances. When a refill is dispensed for a Schedule III or IV substance, the dispensing pharmacist's initials, date the prescription was refilled, and amount of drug dispensed must be documented. Review page 49 of the 2022 version of the DEA Pharmacist's manual for information about the electronic record-keeping of Schedules III–IV refill information.

20 – d

Section 1262 of the Consolidated Appropriations Act of 2023 removes the federal requirement for practitioners to apply for a special waiver ("X" number) prior to prescribing buprenorphine for the treatment of opioid use disorder.

21 – b

Adulteration involves the integrity and composition of a product. If the composition or integrity of a drug is compromised, then the drug is considered adulterated. Some examples of adulteration include:

- A drug contains a decomposed substance

- A drug that is not manufactured under required manufacturing standards

- A drug that is stored in unsanitary conditions

- A substance of the drug container leaches into the drug itself

- A drug that is not pure or contains less than the listed amount of active ingredient

- A drug that contains an unapproved color additive.

22 – d

According to the Code of Federal Regulations, mid-level practitioners are defined as individual practitioners other than physicians, dentists, veterinarians, or podiatrists. Mid-level practitioners include but are not limited to: nurse practitioners, nurse midwives, nurse anesthetists, clinical nurse specialists, physician assistants, optometrists, homeopathic physicians, registered pharmacists, and certified chiropractors.

23 – a, d, e

DME is made for long-term use and must be able to withstand repeated use, be primarily for a medical purpose, and be appropriate for home use. It includes many different types of devices for individuals with a variety of conditions. Some examples of durable medical equipment include wheelchairs, crutches, canes, oxygen, ventilators, and hospital beds.

24 – a

The Prescription Drug Marketing Act (PDMA) of 1987 involves several laws regarding prescription drugs. Primarily, it regulates the storage, distribution, and resale of drug samples. It enforces recordkeeping requirements for prescription drug samples. The PDMA also prohibits hospitals and other health care entities from reselling their drugs to other businesses. This is because hospitals usually obtain drugs at a special rate. Finally, it regulates state licensing of wholesalers.

25 – a, b, c

An NDC number is a numeric, 3-segment code that identifies a drug by manufacturer (first 4 or 5 numbers), specific drug (next 4 numbers), and package (last 2 numbers). NDC numbers are unique to each drug and serve as a universal product identifier for drugs. The expiration date information is not included in the NDC number. By law, the FDA does not require that drug manufacturers include NDC numbers on labels, but it is highly recommended.

NDC numbers are published in an NDC Directory by the FDA. The labeler is responsible for the content of the NDC entry, not the FDA. Therefore, inclusion of information in the NDC directory doesn't mean that the FDA has verified the information. Additionally, assignment of an NDC number does not mean the drug has been approved by the FDA.

26 – a

Isotretinoin is an oral medication used to treat severe acne. Taking isotretinoin during pregnancy can cause birth defects, therefore this drug is highly regulated through a REMS program.

The REMS program for isotretinoin is called iPLEDGE. Under iPLEDGE:

- Only doctors registered with iPLEDGE may prescribe isotretinoin

- Only patients registered with iPLEDGE may receive isotretinoin

- Only pharmacies registered with iPLEDGE may dispense isotretinoin

- Patients may receive no more than a 30-day supply at a time

- No refills are allowed on prescriptions for isotretinoin

- Female patients who can get pregnant must use 2 separate methods of effective birth control 1 month before, while taking, and for 1 month after taking isotretinoin

- Female patients who can get pregnant must take a pregnancy test every month.

27 – b

Compounded drugs cannot be compounded, provided, or sold to other pharmacies or third parties. Compounded drugs cannot be commercially available, must meet national standards, must be a reasonable quantity for current or anticipated prescriptions, and distribution cannot be more than 5% of total prescriptions filled by the pharmacy per year. Drugs that have been removed from the market cannot be used in compounding.

Compounding may be an option to customize medications based upon a doctor's prescription. For example, compounding can customize a drug strength, remove an allergenic component, flavor a medication, and change the dosage form.

28 – b

A DEA Form 222 or an electronically equivalent program is necessary in order to purchase or transfer Schedule II controlled substances.

29 – d

The Schedule II controlled substance prescription can be mailed to the patient. Controlled substances used to not be able to be mailed, but this is no longer the case. The package must contain an inner package with the prescription and appropriate labeling, but must be placed in a plain outer container. The outside package cannot contain information about the contents of the package.

30 – c

Narrow therapeutic index drugs are drugs where small differences in the dose or blood concentration may lead to serious therapeutic failures or adverse reactions. These drugs require careful titration or patient monitoring for safe and effective use. They are permitted to be prescribed.

Some drugs with a narrow therapeutic index are: warfarin, levothyroxine, digoxin, lithium carbonate, phenytoin, and cyclosporine. Additionally, the FDA recommends that potency of the drug have a variability limit of 90% to 105% when the drugs are manufactured.

31 – a

The Poison Prevention Packaging Act (PPPA) set the requirement that prescription drugs, non-prescription drugs, and hazardous household products must have a child-resistant closure. The purpose was to protect children less than 5 years old from poisoning from accidental ingestion or exposure.

Patients may ask to not have safety caps on their medications, especially if they have conditions such as arthritis that make it difficult for them to open up the containers.

There are also several prescription drugs that are exempt from PPPA, such as nitroglycerin sublingual tablets, oral contraceptives in mnemonic dispenser packages, isosorbide dinitrate in sublingual and chewable forms, and more.

32 – a

The Combat Methamphetamine Epidemic Act of 2005 is a federal law that regulates "regulated sellers" including most pharmacies. It sets forth the requirements that these sellers must follow in order to sell ephedrine, pseudoephedrine, and phenylpropanolamine over the counter. Here are some requirements to know:

1) Products must be placed behind the counter or in locked cabinets

2) The identity of the purchasers must be verified, and a log of each sale must be obtained

3) The log must contain:
   - Purchaser's name
   - Address
   - Signature of the purchaser
   - Product sold
   - Quantity sold
   - Date
   - Time

4) The logbook must be kept for 2 years

5) All employees must be trained in the requirements and certify that they have received training

6) The quantity limits are 3.6 grams per day and 9 grams in a 30-day period. No more than 7.5 grams can be imported by mail

7) The logbook requirement does not apply to individual single sales packages of no more than 60 milligrams of pseudoephedrine

The DEA Pharmacist's Manual gives a complete list of proof-of-identity requirements.

33 – a

OTC drug advertising is regulated by the Federal Trade Commission (FTC). Prescription drug advertising is regulated by the Food and Drug Administration (FDA).

34 – c

Under the Drug Supply Chain Security Act, manufacturers are required to provide a transaction report (pedigree) for each product sold. Pharmacies are required to receive this information and pass it along if they further distribute the product. This allows the drugs to be tracked. The transaction report includes 3 parts, also known informally as the "3 T's": transaction information, transaction history, and transaction statement.

35 – e

The Kefauver-Harris Amendment requires that manufacturers provide proof of the effectiveness and safety of their drugs before these drugs can be approved. This was the first "proof-of-efficacy" requirement. The situation that prompted this amendment was the use of thalidomide in Europe that was marketed as a sedative-hypnotic drug that could be used during pregnancy, but it caused serious birth defects. Before the Kefauver-Harris Amendment, the Food, Drug, and Cosmetic Act (FDCA) of 1939 required drugs to be proven safe before being marketed.

36 – c

Pharmacies will use DEA Form 224 to register with the DEA to possess and dispense controlled substances. DEA Form 106 is to report theft or loss of controlled substances. DEA Form 222 to order and transfer Schedule I and II controlled substances. DEA Form 225 is used by manufacturers, distributors, importers, exporters, and researchers to register to conduct business with controlled substances. DEA Form 363 is used by narcotic treatment programs to register to conduct business with controlled substances.

37 – b

A drug product that is manufactured in the U.S., then exported to a foreign country, and then re-imported back to the U.S., is only legal if it is done by the original manufacturer. Re-importation is permitted by the original manufacturer if the purpose is for emergency medical care. Otherwise, re-importation of drugs is not permitted.

Some consumers want to engage in drug re-importation because drugs may be sold at a lower price outside of the United States. It would be a way to obtain access to these lower drug prices from countries such as Canada and Mexico, but it is illegal.

38 – b

Methadone is used for both the treatment of pain (i.e., as an analgesic) and in the detoxification and maintenance of narcotic addiction in patients registered in a narcotic treatment program. While a retail pharmacy may stock methadone, methadone can only be dispensed as an analgesic. Methadone can only be dispensed for the maintenance or detoxification of addicts when it is provided through a registered narcotic treatment center. It can be provided through one of these centers for either short-term detoxification (up to 30 days) or long-term detoxification (30–180 days).

39 – c

The Safe Medical Device Act (SMDA) of 1990 requires health care facilities to report death or injuries caused by or suspected to have been caused by a medical device to the FDA or the manufacturer. The goal is to quickly inform the FDA on the issue so the product can be tracked and potentially recalled for safety reasons. Some examples of medical devices that could be reported are: defibrillators, shunts, lab reagents, pulse oximeters, glucose meters, infusion pumps, wheelchairs, ventilator breathing circuits, needles, and catheters.

40 – c

Misbranding is inaccurate labeling on the drug container. If information is missing, inaccurate, or untrue, this is considered misbranding.

Examples of misbranding include: false or misleading information, unreadable material, omitting a medication guide, inadequate directions or warnings, omitting required information, etc.

41 – a, b, c

According to the Controlled Substances Act, a prescription for a controlled substance must:

1) Be dated and signed on the issue date

2) Include:
   - Patient's full name and address
   - Practitioner's full name, address and DEA number
   - Drug name
   - Drug strength
   - Dosage form
   - Quantity prescribed
   - Directions for use
   - Number of refills authorized
   - Manual signature of the practitioner

3) Be issued for a legitimate medical purpose by a practitioner acting in the usual course of professional practice

4) Not be issued in order for an individual practitioner to obtain a supply of controlled substances to keep on hand for the purpose of general dispensing to patients

Note: Even though the prescriber is responsible for ensuring that the controlled substance prescription is up to the lawful standard, a corresponding responsibility rests with the pharmacist who fills the prescription.

42 – c

A drug (or biologic) is considered to be an orphan drug if it is intended to treat a rare disease or condition that impacts fewer than 200,000 people in the U.S.

Sometimes, an orphan drug designation can be given to drugs citing a cost recovery provision, which is if the cost of research and development of the drug is not reasonably expected to be regained by sales of the drug.

43 – b

Several ingredients such as FD&C Yellow No. 5, aspartame, wintergreen oil, mineral oil, salicylates, sulfites, Ipecac syrup, and alcohol have special labeling requirements under federal regulations. FD&C Yellow No. 5, also called tartrazine, is a color additive that may cause an allergic reaction (itching and hives) in some people. Therefore, a product that contains FD&C Yellow No. 5 must identify so on the label.

44 – e

Normally, a faxed prescription for a Schedule II controlled substance cannot be accepted. However, there are 3 exceptions. Prescriptions for Schedule II controlled substances can be faxed and serve as the original prescription for patients residing in a long-term care facility, enrolled in hospice, or if the drug is to be compounded for direct administration by parenteral, intravenous, intramuscular, subcutaneous, or intraspinal infusion (which includes home infusion therapy).

45 – b

The FDA Adverse Event Reporting System (FAERS) is a database where adverse events from medications can be voluntarily reported. This provides post-marketing safety surveillance on medications.

Meanwhile, the VAERS stands for the Vaccine Adverse Event Reporting System, which is a national vaccine safety surveillance program run by the CDC and FDA.

ERSA, MAERS, and AERS are not drug-related reporting systems.

46 – c

A prescription for a Schedule II controlled substance can be called in orally to be dispensed in an emergency situation. The prescription should be immediately written down by the pharmacist. The quantity should only be enough to adequately cover the emergency period. The pharmacy needs to receive a hard copy prescription from the prescriber within 7 days after authorizing the emergency dispensing. This must also have the words "authorization for emergency dispensing" on the prescription and the date of the oral order written on the front. Prescriptions postmarked within the 7-day period are acceptable. If the prescription is not received in a timely manner, this should be reported to the DEA.

47 – b

The Purple Book contains information related to biological products and information regarding interchangeable biological products. The Orange Book provides information regarding therapeutic equivalence between drugs (excluding biologics). The Red Book is used for drug pricing and packaging information. The Pink Book contains information related to immunizations and vaccine-preventable diseases, as well as information on vaccine safety. Information and recommendation related to international travel (vaccines, diseases, information of other health risks) can be bound in the Yellow Book.

48 – e

An exact count must be made on controlled substances if they are Schedule I or II controlled substances, if they are controlled substances where the bottles contain more than 1000 tablets or capsules, and if the containers are sealed or unopened. Sealed or unopened containers do not need to be opened and counted, but the number marked as the container quantity must be used as an exact count.

49 – b

The U.S. Attorney General, as head of the Justice Department (which the Drug Enforcement Administration is under), may add, delete, or reschedule substances. A scientific and medical recommendation from the Food and Drug Administration is included in the decision.

50 – c

A full NDA must be submitted to the FDA when a manufacturer wants to request reclassification of a current prescription-only drug to be an over-the-counter drug. This is just one method of requesting reclassification, as there are four different methods. Another method is the FDA granting an exemption if determining prescription-only status is not necessary for the safety and protection of the public. A third method is filing a supplement to the original NDA (a "supplemental NDA") for review of the drug's safety and adverse events. The last method is if the Nonprescription Drug Advisory Committee recommends the ingredient contained in the drug be converted to a non-prescription status.

An ANDA is an application for the potential approval of a generic drug product. Both EIND and IND are applications regarding the development of a new drug. A marketed new drug application is not an existing type of application.

51 – a

In order to verify a DEA number, use the following process:

1) Add together the first, third, and fifth numbers.

2) Add together the second, fourth, and sixth numbers. Multiply this number by two.

3) Add the numbers together from steps 1 and 2. The last digit of the number you get from step 3 is the last number of the DEA number.

Using the DEA number BS5927683, the process would be:

1) 5 + 2 + 6 = 13

2) (9 + 7 + 8) × 2 = (24) × 2 = 48

3) 13 + 48 = 61 → Since the last digit is 1, the DEA should end in 1, not 3.

52 – d

Dentists must prescribe within their scope of practice. Accordingly, prescriptions written by a dentist must treat a disease of the mouth, treat discomfort of the mouth, or be used to facilitate a dental procedure. Atorvastatin is used to lower cholesterol. Other professions, such as optometrists and veterinarians, must also prescribe within their scope of practice.

53 – e

A DEA Form 222 must be signed and dated by the person authorized to sign the pharmacy's DEA registration. This means that only the pharmacist who signed the most recent application for renewal of the pharmacy's DEA registration may sign a DEA Form 222. Additionally, that pharmacist may authorize others to sign a DEA Form 222 by granting a power of attorney. A power of attorney must be signed by the registrant (the person granting the power), the person to whom the power of attorney is being granted, and two witnesses.

54 – b

Phase 1 clinical trials are conducted in a small group of healthy participants without the disease condition. Typically, the study size is around 20–80 people. The goal of the Phase 1 clinical trial is to study the properties of the drug and determine safety. Sometimes the Phase 1 clinical trial can include participants with the disease condition, but this is not as common.

Phase 2 clinical trials are conducted in a larger size group of 100 or more people, and these participants have the disease condition. Phase 2 clinical trials study the effectiveness of the drug.

Phase 3 clinical trials are conducted in a larger group of hundreds or thousands of participants who have the disease condition. The drug's safety, efficacy, and dosing are further studied. If a drug passes the Phase 3 study, then it can be approved by the FDA.

Finally, Phase 4 clinical trials are conducted after the drug is approved and looks at the safety and efficacy of the drug long-term, also called post-marketing surveillance.

55 – c

A pharmacy may keep shipping and financial data for controlled substances at a central location other than the registered location after notifying the nearest DEA Diversion Field Office. Executed DEA Form 222 orders, controlled substance prescriptions, and controlled substance inventories must be kept at the pharmacy location that is registered with the DEA and cannot be kept at a central location.

56 – c

Schedule III controlled substances have less potential for abuse than Schedule I or II drugs, and they have a currently accepted medical use in the U.S. Codeine by itself is classified under Schedule II, but in combination with acetaminophen it is a Schedule III drug.

57 – e

HIPAA permits the use of protected health information (PHI) for treatment purposes. Medical information can be shared to persons involved in the patient's care without written or verbal consent.

58 – b

The Federal Transfer Warning ("Caution: Federal law prohibits the transfer of this drug to any person other than the patient for whom it was prescribed") is required on the label of Schedule II–IV controlled substances when dispensed to a patient. Most pharmacies comply with this requirement by including this warning on all prescription labels. However, it is not legally required on prescription labels for Schedule V controlled substances and non-controlled prescriptions.

59 – a

Outsourcing facilities, also known as 503B facilities, are permitted to compound sterile products without receiving patient-specific prescriptions or medication orders. They are regulated by the FDA and subject to current good manufacturing practices. Compounded products must be distributed within a health care setting or dispensed directly to a patient or prescriber, and may not be sold or transferred to a wholesaler for redistribution.

A pharmacy that registers as an outsourcing facility would therefore be able to compound sterile products without receiving patient-specific prescriptions.

60 – b, c, e

The Health Information Technology for Economic and Clinical Health Act (HITECH Act) promotes health information technology to advance healthcare and the use of electronic health records. The HIPAA Breach Notification Rule is a part of this act.

It requires entities to notify affected individuals without unreasonable delay, and in no case later than 60 days following the discovery of a breach of unsecured protected health information. Breaches of 500 or more records also need to be reported to the Secretary of the U.S. Department of Health and Human Services (HHS) within 60 days of the discovery of the breach, and smaller breaches within 60 days of the end of the calendar year in which the breach occurred. In addition to reporting the breach to the HHS Secretary, a notice of a breach of 500 or more records must be provided to prominent media outlets serving the state or jurisdiction affected by the breach.

61 – d

The USP Chapter <797> describes the requirements of sterile compounded preparations, including responsibilities of compounding personnel, training, facilities, environmental monitoring, and storage and testing. USP Chapter <795> covers nonsterile compounding, and USP Chapter <800> describes safe handling of hazardous drugs. USP <503A> and USP <503B> do not exist as USP chapters; however, the terms 503A and 503B are used to designate compounding pharmacies.

62 – b, c, d

Every person or firm that manufactures, distributes, or dispenses any controlled substance must register with the DEA. However, patients who receive controlled substance prescriptions and pharmacists working in a pharmacy are exempt from DEA registration requirements. Therefore, pharmacists do not need to have a DEA number to dispense controlled substances.

63 – b

Clozapine is associated with severe neutropenia, which can lead to severe infections. Prescribers are required to be certified in the clozapine REMS program before prescribing clozapine. Pharmacies are also required to be certified in the clozapine REMS program to dispense clozapine.

64 – c

A DEA Form 41 is used to document the destruction of controlled substances. More commonly, a pharmacy will transfer controlled substances to an authorized reverse distributor for destruction. The reverse distributor then fills out DEA Form 41 to document the destruction of controlled substances.

65 – b

The Federal Anti-Tampering Act requires tamper-evident packaging of many over-the-counter products and cosmetics to avoid contamination issues and limit access. If the items were tampered with, it would be evident due to the packaging of these products. For example, some products have a tamper-evident closure cap, tamper-evident liner, and tamper-evident tape. The act was passed in response to the Tylenol poisoning deaths in Chicago in 1982, where the Tylenol capsules were contaminated with cyanide.

66 – a

Schedule I controlled substances include drugs that have a high potential for abuse and severe potential for dependence, with no currently accepted medical use in the U.S. This includes heroin, lysergic acid diethylamide (LSD), mescaline, and methaqualone, among others.

67 – c

Manufacturer's containers of OTC medications are required to display the following information: identity of the product (active ingredient), inactive ingredient(s), purpose, use(s), warnings, directions, and storage information.

Other information that is not required, but may be included, is as follows: net quantity of contents, name and address of the manufacturer/packager/distributor, lot number or batch code, expiration date, and instructions for what to do if an overdose occurs.

While the Poison Control Center phone number is included on some OTC medications, it is not required by federal law.

68 – b

Patient Package Inserts (PPIs) must be provided to patients in acute-care hospitals or long-term care facilities prior to the first administration and every 30 days thereafter. They are required for oral contraceptives and estrogen-containing products.

69 – c

DEA registration permits pharmacies, manufacturers, distributors, importers, exporters, and researchers to possess controlled substances. A DEA registration is valid for 36 months. Registrants will receive renewal notification approximately 60 days prior to the DEA registration expiration date.

70 – c

For recordkeeping requirements, executed copies of DEA Form 222 must be maintained separately from all other records. If a pharmacy stores these forms electronically, then the electronic records are deemed separate if such copies are readily retrievable from all other electronic records. A defective DEA Form 222 cannot be corrected and needs to be replaced by a new form. Finally, when filling out the DEA Form 222, only 1 item may be entered on each numbered line.

71 – e

Under the Health Insurance Portability and Accountability Act (HIPAA) Privacy Rule, a communication is not considered "marketing" if it is made for the treatment of the individual. Therefore, refill reminders for currently prescribed medications (or one that has not lapsed for more than 90 days) are not considered marketing. Therefore, offering this service is not a HIPAA violation. Patients may be charged for this service as long as any payment made to the pharmacy is reasonable and related to the pharmacy's cost of making the communication. Mailed refill reminders are valid, as well as electronic refill reminders.

As a note, the HIPAA Privacy Rule defines marketing as making "a communication about a product or service that encourages recipients of the communication to purchase or use the product or service." An entity would need to receive authorization from the patient to send out marketing communications.

72 – d

Manufacturer's expiration dates may be expressed as a day, month, and year, or as just a month and year. If it is written as only month and year, the drug expires on the last day of the listed month. The drug is safe to use on the expiration date, but not after.

73 – c

A prospective DUR consists of reviewing a prescription for adverse effects, therapeutic duplication, drug-disease interactions and contraindications, drug dosing and regimen, drug allergies, clinical misuse or abuse, drug interactions, medication appropriateness, overutilization, underutilization, and pregnancy alerts. Ensuring compliance with prescription labeling is not part of the prospective DUR.

74 – a

The purpose of the Federal Hazardous Substances Act (FHSA) is to protect consumers from hazardous or toxic substances. The FHSA requires precautionary labeling on the immediate container of hazardous household products, which includes certain OTC medications. Medication packages would include the statement, "Keep out of the reach of children." Depending on the hazardous substance, additional warnings and statements, such as "handle with gloves" or "harmful if swallowed," may be required. The warning "Keep out of the reach of children" applies to OTC drugs and not FDA-regulated drugs.

75 – c

The 5% rule states that a pharmacy does not have to register with the DEA as a distributor if the total quantity of controlled substances distributed during a 12-month period does not exceed 5% of the total quantity of all controlled substances dispensed and distributed during that period.

76 – d

The Occupational and Safety Health Administration (OSHA) requires that employers meet the Hazardous Communication Standard. This includes having a Hazardous Communication Plan, which lists hazardous chemicals in the workplace, and ensuring that all such products are appropriately labeled and have a Safety Data Sheet. Workers must be trained on the hazards of chemicals, appropriate protective measures, and where to find more information. The purpose of OSHA is to protect employees, which is separate from laws intended to protect consumers and patients.

77 – b

The Consumer Product Safety Commission administers the Poison Prevention Packaging Act (PPPA). This act requires child-resistant containers for all prescriptions and certain non-prescription drugs, unless there is an exemption for a specific drug or circumstance.

78 – d

Bulk compounding of products in order to sell them to other pharmacies is considered "manufacturing," which is regulated by the FDA. Note that for manufacturing, a patient-specific prescription is not required. So, in this case, since there is not a patient-specific prescription involved, the mass production of ibuprofen suppositories is considered manufacturing. On the other hand, "compounding" is typically regulated by state boards of pharmacy and is limited to compounding prescriptions for individual patients pursuant to a prescription.

79 – e

The Prescription Drug Marketing Act bans most pharmacies from purchasing, trading, selling, or possessing prescription drug samples. The only exception is for pharmacies that are owned by a charitable organization or by a city, state, or county government and that are part of a health care entity providing care to indigent or low-income patients at no or reduced cost. In this case, samples may only be provided at no cost to the patients.

80 – e

DEA Form 222 is used to transfer and order Schedule II controlled substances. The DEA used to allow this form to be faxed, but not anymore. A DEA Form 224 is needed for a pharmacy to dispense controlled substances. Schedule III–V controlled substances may be ordered through normal ordering processes from wholesalers or manufacturers, but must be documented by the pharmacy with an invoice upon receipt. The common term used for ordering Schedule III–V controlled substances is "using an invoice."

81 – d

Manufacturers and packagers of over-the-counter drugs for sale at retail must package products in tamper-evident packaging, with some exceptions. The exceptions are dermatological, dentifrice, insulin, or lozenge products.

82 – c

A pharmacist may not change the following items on a Schedule II controlled substance prescription: name of the patient, name of the drug, and name of the prescriber. All other information, including quantity, directions for use, drug strength, and dosage form, may be changed with the verbal permission of the prescriber as long as the change is documented on the prescription.

83 – e

Patients have a right to obtain a copy of their protected health information. Pharmacies must comply with such a request within 30 days. If there is a delay, the patient must be notified of the reason for delay and the pharmacy may extend the time by no more than 30 additional days. Normally, pharmacies are able to give a copy of the prescription record on the day of the request.

84 - b

Thalidomide is an immunomodulatory agent as well as a chemotherapy drug. Thalidomide causes a high frequency of birth defects in pregnant females. Babies were born with missing or deformed arms and legs. Therefore, the REMS program was developed to ensure safe use and monitoring of thalidomide.

85 – c

The Kefauver-Harris Amendment of 1962 is more commonly known as the "Drug Efficacy Amendment." It requires new drugs to be proven as safe and effective before they are approved. It also allows the FDA to establish good drug manufacturing practices and gives the FDA jurisdiction over prescription drug advertising, which must include accurate information about side effects. It also controls the marketing of generic drugs to keep them from being sold as expensive medications under new trade names.

86 – c

Anabolic steroids are classified as Schedule III controlled substances under federal law. An example of an anabolic steroid is testosterone.

87 – d

The Durham-Humphrey Amendment created two separate categories of drugs, prescription (legend) and over-the-counter (OTC). Prescription drugs require a prescription and must be dispensed under medical supervision. OTC drugs can be obtained without a prescription and do not require medical supervision.

88 – d

Generic bioequivalence information is found in the FDA Orange Book. A two-letter coding system indicates equivalency, with the first letter being key. Codes that start with the letter A indicate that the FDA considers the drug products to be pharmaceutically and therapeutically equivalent. Codes that start with the letter B indicate that the FDA does not consider the products to be equivalent.

The second letter of the code typically indicates the dosage form (for example, a code of AT would indicate that two topical products are equivalent).

Products with known or potential equivalency issues, but for which adequate scientific evidence exists to establish bioequivalence, are given a code of AB.

89 – a, b, d

DEA registration is not required for an agent or employee of any registered manufacturer, distributor, or dispenser if acting in the usual course of business. This includes pharmacists working at pharmacies and nurses working in a hospital or physician's office. Patients who possess controlled substances for a lawful purpose are not required to register with the DEA.

Providers must register with the DEA unless practicing under the registration of a hospital or other institution. Each pharmacy must have its own DEA registration to dispense controlled substances.

90 – d

A product is considered adulterated if its strength or quality differs from what it represents (this is not the only criteria for adulteration, but one example). A product is misbranded if the labeling is false or misleading. If a drug product's strength is less than what is represented on the label, then the drug product is considered both adulterated and misbranded.

91 – d

Patients may request easy-open containers (containers that are not child-resistant) for any prescription. A provider may also make this request on a patient's behalf (written or verbal), but can only do so for one individual prescription. Only a patient can issue a blanket request for easy-open containers on all future prescriptions. There is not a legal requirement for documentation of easy-open container requests, but it is good practice for a pharmacist to have documentation in case an issue arises.

92 – c

Risk Evaluation and Mitigation Strategies (REMS) are strategies to manage a known or potential serious risk associated with a drug. A REMS program does not have anything to do with the affordability of drugs.

93 – c

Federal regulations require a warning statement, including a warning about the risk of Reye's syndrome in children, on aspirin and other salicylate products. An example warning statement is: "Keep out of reach of children. In case of overdose, get medical help or contact a Poison Control Center right away." Containers of chewable 81mg (1.25 grain) aspirin may not contain more than 36 tablets in order to reduce the risk of accidental poisoning in children. In other words, if a child were to open a bottle of aspirin and ingest all 36 tablets, 36 tablets would generally be considered a non-toxic amount.

94 – b

DEA registration numbers begin with two letters. The first letter indicates practitioner status, in which "M" is the designation for mid-level practitioners. The second letter typically indicates the first letter of the practitioner's last name, the first letter of the pharmacy name, or the first letter of the hospital name.

To verify the DEA registration number, first add together the 1st, 3rd, and 5th digit. Then add together the 2nd, 4th, and 6th digit, and multiply this number by two. Add these two numbers together. The last digit (in the ones place) of the sum of these two numbers should match the last number of the DEA registration number.

Check each of the five choices. For the second choice (MT1200980):

1) $1 + 0 + 9 = 10$

2) $2 + 0 + 8 = 10$; $10 \times 2 = 20$

3) $10 + 20 = 30$

The last digit of 30 is 0, so 0 must be the last digit of the DEA number: MT1200980.

95 – a, b, d

The FDA requires medication guides be issued with certain prescription drugs and biologics if they determine the drug has serious risks relative to benefits, when patient adherence is crucial to the effectiveness of the drug, when there is a known serious side effect, and when providing information can prevent serious adverse effects. Medication guides do not replace pharmacist counseling. A patient also does not need to be in a nursing home to receive a medication guide. Some drugs which require a guide be dispensed with each fill are: aripiprazole, amphetamine/dextroamphetamine, fentanyl, testosterone, citalopram, ciprofloxacin, amiodarone, duloxetine, adalimumab, and more.

96 – e

Omnibus Budget Reconciliation Act of 1990 (commonly known as OBRA 90) set the requirement that patients must be offered counseling on medications. Patients have the right to refuse this counseling, but counseling must at least be offered.

97 – a, b, e

Several drugs are exempt from the child-resistant container packaging requirement. Some examples include sublingual nitroglycerin tablets, methylprednisolone tablets containing no more than 84mg per package, preparations in aerosol containers intended for inhalation, and more. Effervescent aspirin or acetaminophen tablets are exempt, but non-effervescent tablets are not. Packages of prednisone tablets are only exempt if they contain less than 105mg per package.

98 – b

Prescription records are required to be kept for a minimum of 2 years based on federal law. However, if there are stricter state laws, those should be followed. For example, if a state requires prescription records to be maintained for 5 years, then prescription records must be maintained for at least 5 years because it is stricter than 2 years.

99 – b

Aripiprazole (Abilify) is a drug that has a medication guide. Drugs that pose a serious or significant concern have medication guides. The medication guide is required for each dispensing, including refills. The medication guide is required as part of the labeling. If the medication guide is not given, the drug is considered misbranded.

100 – b

CMS regulations require a consultant pharmacist to perform a drug regimen review for long-term care patients at least once a month.

Answer Index — Florida Questions

1 – d

The Governor appoints the Board of Pharmacy members. These appointments are confirmed by the Senate.

2 – d

A practitioner may dispense no more than a 14-day supply of a Schedule III medication in the legal course of his/her practice for a surgical procedure. For Schedule II opioids, they may dispense no more than a 3-day supply, or up to a 7-day supply if certain criteria are met.

3 – c

The Florida Board of Pharmacy consists of 9 members.

4 – d

Expiration dates written by month and year expire on the last day of the month.

5 – e

The Drug Wholesale Distributor Advisory Council consists of 12 members. The Secretary of Business and Professional Regulation (or a designee) and the Secretary of Health Care Administration (or a designee) are two members of the Council that appoint 10 other members. The other members must consist of: 3 persons employed by a different national primary wholesale distributor, 1 person employed by retail pharmacy chain, 1 hospital pharmacist, 1 person employed by a secondary wholesale distributor, 1 person from the Board of Pharmacy, 1 physician, 1 person employed by a pharmaceutical manufacturer, and 1 person employed by a medical gas manufacturer or wholesaler.

6 – c

The Board of Pharmacy consists of seven pharmacists who are practicing in the state of Florida. These pharmacists must also represent certain practice settings.

7 – b, c, e

An emergency oral prescription for a Schedule II controlled substance may be issued when immediate administration of the drug is necessary for proper treatment, the prescriber is unable to issue a written prescription at the time, and there is no alternative treatment available.

8 – d

Each pharmacy must have a CQI committee that meets once every 3 months.

9 – e

In order to be registered in the state of Florida as a non-resident pharmacy, the pharmacy must be open for a minimum of 40 hours per week.

10 – d

The following drugs are on the negative drug formulary: digitoxin, conjugated estrogen, dicumarol, chlorpromazine (solid oral dosage forms), theophylline (controlled release), and pancrelipase (oral dosage forms). Premarin is a conjugated estrogen.

11 – c

Although drugs cannot be used past the expiration date, it is not the only limitation. Unclaimed prescriptions can be reused for dispensing in a pharmacy for a period of up to one year from the fill date unless it expires sooner or if it is recalled.

12 – b

There must be at least two witnesses present for the destruction of controlled substances at an institutional Class I pharmacy nursing home.

13 – e

Nurse practitioners may prescribe non-controlled substances and Schedule II–V controlled substances as long as it is in their protocol.

14 – a, b, c, d, e

A pharmacist who receives a prescription for a brand name drug shall, unless requested otherwise by the purchaser, substitute a less expensive, generically equivalent drug. The pharmacist must notify the person presenting the prescription of the substitution, of the retail price difference between the brand name drug and the generic, and that the person presenting may refuse the substitution.

A substitution should not be made if the prescriber indicates that the brand name drug is medically necessary.

15 – a

At least two of the seven pharmacists on the Board of Pharmacy must be community pharmacists.

16 – a

A copy of the completed and witnessed Form DEA 41 must be mailed to the DEA within 1 business day after the destruction of the drugs.

In lieu of destruction on the premises, controlled substances may also be shipped to reverse distributors for destruction in conformity with federal guidelines.

17 – b

The permittee must notify the Florida Board of Pharmacy within fourteen days of receiving the pharmacy permit that the opening and operation of the pharmacy will be delayed.

18 – e

At least one member of the board must be 60 years of age or older.

19 – b

A backup copy of information from pharmacy data processing systems must be kept and updated at least once weekly.

20 – d

A pharmacy intern must complete a 20-hour immunization program for vaccine administration in order to become certified to administer vaccinations.

21 – b

Thirty hours (3 C.E.U.s) of approved continuing education are required within the two years prior to license renewal.

22 – a

A prescription can be transferred to a pharmacy that is out of the state of Florida, but it is the responsibility of the transferring pharmacist to verify the transfer is going to a licensed pharmacist and pharmacy.

23 – c

A pharmacist must be allowed at least 10 days to produce documentation to address any discrepancies found during a Medicaid audit.

24 – c

The closest DEA field office must be notified within 14 days before the proposed date of the transfer of pharmacy ownership.

25 – d

All controlled substances (Schedule II–V) may be prescribed electronically. The electronic prescribing system must be Board-approved.

26 – a

The baseline rule allows for a ratio of 1:1. However, meeting certain criteria allows for ratios of 1:3, 1:6, or 1:8 (pharmacist:technician).

27 – b

Members of the Board of Pharmacy serve 4-year terms. As the terms come to an end, a new member will be appointed.

28 – b, d, e

Information that must be documented when Schedule III–V controlled substances are transferred to a new pharmacy includes: the pharmacy names, addresses, and DEA registration numbers; the drug name, dosage form, and quantity; the date transferred.

29 – d

Modified Class II institutional pharmacies must establish a Pharmacy Services Committee that must meet at least once annually.

30 – a

A customized medication package is a package that is prepared by a pharmacist for a specific patient. It is a series of containers with two or more solid oral dosage forms.

31 – a

Twenty hours (2 C.E.U.s) of approved continuing education are required to be completed every two years by pharmacy technicians.

32 – b

Four hours of the twenty continuing education hours required every two years for pharmacy technicians must be completed via live presentation.

33 – c

Within 7 days after authorizing an emergency oral prescription, the prescriber must have a written prescription for the quantity prescribed delivered to the dispensing pharmacist.

34 – c

The pharmacy permit must be returned to the Board of Pharmacy within 10 days after the closing of a pharmacy.

35 – a

Two hours of the total of twenty continuing education hours every two years must be related to prevention of medication errors and pharmacy law.

36 – e

A pharmacist can administer a long-acting antipsychotic when there is a protocol established with a physician and they receive a separate prescription for each injection. The pharmacist must also follow regulations regarding safe disposal of medication and injection waste. A continuing education course must be completed before being able to administer long-acting antipsychotics.

37 – c

Prescription records must be kept for 4 years after the creation or receipt of the records.

38 – a

A pharmacy technician must obtain at least one hour of continuing education on HIV/AIDS before the first license renewal.

39 – d

Schedule V controlled substance quantities sold to any one individual within a 48-hour period are limited to 240 milligrams of opium.

40 – e

A prescription filled at a central fill pharmacy must have both the originating pharmacy and central fill pharmacy identified on the prescription label. The central fill pharmacy may be identified by a code, but the originating pharmacy should be identified by name and address.

41 – a, b, c

When destroying controlled substances at an institutional Class I pharmacy nursing home, there must be at least two witnesses. Witnesses must be facility administrators, directors of nursing, consultant pharmacists, sworn law enforcement officers, or licensed physicians, mid-level practitioners, nurses, or other pharmacists employed by or under contract or written agreement with the facility.

42 – d

Pharmacists must attempt to make sure there is a reasonable effort to obtain such information for a patient profile at the pharmacy: patient name, address, phone number, date of birth, gender, chronic diseases, comprehensive list of medications and relevant devices, known allergies and drug interactions, and any other relevant information for counseling.

43 – d

Number of refills are not required to be on the label. Requirements for drug labels are: name and address of the dispensing pharmacy, patient name, prescriber name, date of dispensing, prescription number, drug dispensed, directions for use, expiration date or beyond-use-date. For controlled substances, a warning that it is a crime to transfer the substance to any person other than the patient must be included.

44 – d

A prospective drug review consists of reviewing at least the known allergies, reasonable dose and duration, therapeutic duplication, drug interactions (drug-drug, drug-disease), and proper drug utilization (abuse or misuse). This does not mean cost-effective alternatives cannot be reviewed, but they are not a necessary part of a review.

45 – b

A customized patient medication package is where there are multi-dose units physically connected or in a connected container.

46 – d

After a change in prescription department manager, an internet pharmacy must notify the Board of Pharmacy within 30 days.

47 – c

Schedule II controlled substances may be partially filled if the pharmacist is unable to fill the entire portion of the prescription. The remaining portion must be filled within 72 hours of the original dispensing; otherwise, the prescribing practitioner will have to be notified and more could only be dispensed upon receiving a new prescription.

48 – c

Consultant pharmacists that have ordering labs or clinical testing as part of their job authority must have 3 hours of continuing education relating to ordering lab and clinical tests within the two years before license renewal.

49 – d

Pharmacies located outside of the state of Florida that deliver prescriptions to residents of Florida in any manner must be registered with the state of Florida. Non-resident pharmacies must notify the Florida Board of Pharmacy within 30 days of a change in the prescription department manager or corporate officer.

50 – e

Schedule II medications can typically only be dispensed based on a written prescription. In the case of emergency situations, an oral prescription can be used to dispense a Schedule II medication. It must be limited to a 72-hour supply.

51 – a

A Class I institutional pharmacy administers medications from individual prescription containers to individual patients and they do not dispense medications.

52 – c

A Class II institutional pharmacy has registered pharmacists providing dispensing and consulting services on institution premises to the patients of the institution. A Modified Class II institutional pharmacy is at a short-term primary care treatment center.

53 – a

Certain medicinal drugs can be ordered and dispensed by the pharmacist with a limited days' supply. Urinary analgesics, such as phenazopyridine, can be ordered for up to a 2-day supply. Some others include otic analgesics (antipyrine, benzocaine, glycerin), anti-nausea preparations (meclizine, scopolamine), antihistamines and decongestants for patients older than 6 years, topical and otic antifungal and antibacterial agents, topical anti-inflammatory agents, keratolytics, vitamins with fluoride, medicinal shampoos, ophthalmics, histamine H2 antagonists, benzoyl peroxide for acne, topical antivirals (acyclovir, penciclovir). These other categories of medications have certain stipulations upon ordering and dispensing that can be found in Florida Administrative Code 64B16-27.220.

54 – a, c, d

When a medication is dispensed in the manufacturer's package, it must bear a label with the practitioner's name, patient's name, and date of dispensing.

55 – e

A Modified Class II institutional pharmacy still meets the requirements of a Class II institutional pharmacy other than space and equipment requirements.

56 – d

Any known or believed attempts to fraudulently obtain a controlled substance must be reported to the law enforcement agency or sheriff by the pharmacist by the end of the next business day or within 24 hours, whichever is later. If the pharmacist fails to report, it is considered a misdemeanor of the first degree.

57 – a

Medicaid audits are to be conducted by a pharmacist licensed in the state of Florida.

58 – e

An internet pharmacy in the state of Florida must be open for a minimum 40 hours per week.

59 – b

After a change in responsible person, specialty pharmacies must notify the Board of Pharmacy within 10 days.

60 – a

An open formulary is where an institution can stock/purchase/prescribe any drug without prior approval from the medical staff or supervisors. The inventory may be kept on supply and demand.

61 – b

The Florida Board of Pharmacy must have at least 2 public representatives serving on the Board that are in no way connected to the profession of pharmacy.

62 – c

Vaccine administration records must be kept for a minimum of 5 years.

63 – d

A pharmacist must maintain at least $200,000 of professional liability insurance and the completion of vaccine administration training in order to enter into a protocol for vaccine administration.

64 – a, b, e

Some new substances that are created are not controlled, but may have "potential for abuse." A substance is considered to have "potential for abuse" if it has properties that create a substantial likelihood of being: taken per the user's own initiative rather than based on how prescribed, used in amounts that are hazardous to the user's health or community safety, or are diverted from legal use or distributed illegally.

65 – a, c, d

All controlled substance prescriptions must include: date of issuance, name of the prescriber, address of the prescriber, DEA number of the prescriber, prescriber signature, full name and address of the patient, drug name and strength, dosage form, quantity to dispense, and directions for use.

66 – b

Up to 5 continuing education hours per two-year license renewal period can be obtained through volunteering in an area of critical need, or serving the indigent or underserved populations. However, the order to receive credit for this volunteer work must be submitted prior to volunteering and receive approval from the Board.

67 – d

A pharmacy technician applicant must complete at least 1500 hours of an apprenticeship under the supervision of a Florida registered pharmacist if seeking technician status through means of an apprenticeship. Otherwise, a technician applicant can complete an instructional program or certification through a nationally accredited program.

68 – c

The agency conducting the pharmacy records audit must give the pharmacist a 7-day notice before the initial audit of the cycle. This applies for audits done by a managed care company, insurance company, third-party payor, pharmacy benefit manager, or other entity that represents such parties.

69 – a

Physicians, authorized physician assistants, nurse practitioners, and veterinarians may administer or prescribe Schedule II controlled substances. In the case of veterinarians, this may only be done for the treatment of animals. Optometrists may not administer or prescribe a Schedule II controlled substance.

70 – d

Such prescribing and dispensing must be for a supply of the drug that will last for the greater of the following:

Up to 48 hours; or
Through the end of the next business day.

71 – e

The first letter for a physician will always be A, B, F, or G. The second letter must be the first letter of the physician's last name. To determine if the numbers in the DEA number are valid, the first, third, and fifth numbers should be added. Then, the second, fourth, and sixth numbers should be added and multiplied by 2. The sum of the first set of numbers and that of the second (multiplied by 2) should then be added. The last digit of the answer should be the last digit of the DEA number. The first letters of M and P and the second letter R eliminates three answer choices. Check the others to find that AT3851424 works:

$3 + 5 + 4 = 12$
$(8 + 1 + 2) \times 2 = 22$

Adding those up gives: $12 + 22 = 34$
So, the last digit of the DEA number would be 4.

72 – d

Schedule III–V medications may not be refilled more than 5 times within a 6-month period from the date written.

73 – d

The Board of Pharmacy must be notified in writing within 20 days of the commencement or cessation of pharmacy practice in the state of Florida when it was a result of pending or completed disciplinary action.

74 – c

A pharmacist cannot dispense more than a 30-day supply of a Schedule III medication that is received as an oral prescription.

75 – b

The agency conducting the Medicaid audit must give the pharmacist a 1-week notice before the initial audit of the cycle.

76 – a, b, c, d

Upon receiving a transferred prescription, before dispensing the medication, certain information must be recorded in writing or by electronic means: prescription order, name of transferring pharmacy, prescription number, name of the drug, the original amount dispensed, date of original dispensing, and the number of remaining authorized refills.

77 – d

A pharmacist may dispense a one-time emergency refill of up to a 72-hour supply of any medication that is not a Schedule II medication or up to one vial of insulin for diabetes.

78 – b

The pharmacy owner must contact the Board of Pharmacy and local DEA office within 24 hours of discovering the damage due to weather or another disaster. This should be done in writing.

79 – b

After a change in responsible person, nuclear pharmacies must notify the Board of Pharmacy within 10 days.

80 – c

Schedule V controlled substance quantities sold to any one individual within a 48-hour period are limited to 120 milligrams of codeine.

81 – e

A written prescription for a controlled substance must have the quantity prescribed in both textual and numerical formats.

82 – c

The storage, compounding, dispensing, and Hot lab area of a nuclear pharmacy must be at least 150 square feet.

83 – a

An institutional pharmacy may only have medication samples upon written request from the prescribing practitioner.

84 – b

An onsite audit can only be scheduled after the first 3 calendar days of a month when being audited by a managed care company, insurance company, third-party payor, pharmacy benefit manager, or other entity that represents such parties. An audit can only be done earlier if the pharmacist consents otherwise.

85 – d

If the Governor issues an emergency order or proclamation of a state of emergency, a pharmacist may dispense an emergency refill of up to a 30-day supply. This does not apply to Schedule II drugs. The medication must be essential to the maintenance of life or to the continuation of therapy in a chronic condition. The pharmacist must also use professional judgment to determine that the interruption of therapy might reasonably produce undesirable health consequences or may cause physical or mental discomfort. They must create and sign a written order containing all of the required prescription information and must notify the prescriber of the emergency dispensing within a reasonable time period.

86 – b, c, e

Class II institutional pharmacy policy and procedures manuals must contain information regarding each pharmacist working with remote medication order processing. Their information should include their name, address, phone number, and license number.

87 – d

The license renewal date for immunization certificate licenses is September 30th.

88 – c

Five hours of continuing education may be obtained in risk management through attending one full day or 8 hours of a disciplinary Board of Pharmacy meeting. The pharmacist must remain in continuous attendance and must not be part of a hearing. Pharmacists attending must sign in with the Board designee or Executive Director.

89 – b, c, e

When a pharmacy is contacted to request a transfer to a different pharmacy, along with providing all necessary information for a transfer and recording "void" on the prescription, the name of the requesting pharmacy and pharmacist and the date of transfer request must be recorded on the prescription.

90 – c, e

One option is to have it witnessed and signed by the prescription department manager or the consultant pharmacist of record along with a D.E.A. agent, or a Department inspector. Another option is the prescription department manager or the consultant pharmacist of record along with one of the following: medical director or his/her physician designee, director of nursing or his/her licensed nurse designee, or a sworn law enforcement officer.

91 – b, c, d, e

A counterfeit-proof prescription pad must contain the following security features: the background color must be blue or green and resist reproduction; the pad must be printed on artificial watermarked paper; the pad must resist erasures and alterations; and the word "void" or "illegal" must appear on any photocopy or other reproduction of the pad.

92 – c

At least two of the seven pharmacists on the Board must work in Class II or Modified Class II institutional pharmacies. Two others must be community pharmacists, and the remaining three can work in any practice setting as long as they are actively practicing.

93 – a, d, e

Drugs dispensed by a practitioner in the legal course of his/her practice that are not dispensed in the manufacturer's bottle must have a label containing: the practitioner's name, patient's name, date of dispensing, name and strength of drug, and directions for use. When a medication is dispensed in the manufacturer's package, it must bear a label with the practitioner's name, patient's name, and date of dispensing.

94 – c

A registered intern or registered pharmacy technician who administers an immunization or vaccine must be supervised by a certified pharmacist at a ratio of one pharmacist to a maximum of five registered interns or registered pharmacy technicians, or a combination thereof.

95 – e

Nurse practitioners may not prescribe psychotropic drugs to patients under the age of 18.

96 – c

Certain medicinal drugs can be ordered and dispensed by the pharmacist with a limited day supply. Oral analgesics can be ordered for mild to moderate pain for up to a 6-day supply.

97 – a

Two hours of the total of 30 continuing education hours every two years must be related to medication errors.

98 – c

E-FORCSE (Electronic Florida Online Reporting of Controlled Substance Evaluation Program) is the PDMP used in the state of Florida.

99 – e

Registered pharmacists must complete a total of 10 continuing education hours by live presentation, live video teleconference, or interactive computer-based application every two years.

100 – c

Medications filled at a Class II institutional central fill pharmacy may only be delivered to the originating pharmacy.

101 – a

Pharmacists must complete two hours of board-approved continuing education on validating of prescriptions for controlled substances every two years before license renewal.

102 – a

Doctors of Medicine, Osteopathy, Dental Surgery, Dental Medicine, Podiatric Medicine, Veterinary Medicine, Physician Assistants, Advanced Registered Nurse Practitioners, and Naturopaths can prescribe therapeutic drugs within their scope of practice. Certified optometrists and pharmacists have limited prescribing authority as well.

103 – b

Schedule V controlled substance quantities sold to any one individual within a 48-hour period are limited to 60 milligrams of dihydrocodeine.

104 – b

Any pharmacist that has a retired license for more than 5 years or has not been active in the state of Florida must take and pass both the jurisprudence exam and the NAPLEX. If a pharmacist has been retired for less than 5 years, they would only have to take the jurisprudence exam.

105 – d

A pharmacist must complete an 8-hour continuing education course regarding the safe and effective administration of behavioral health and antipsychotic injections. The continuing education must be offered by an accredited statewide professional association of physicians in Florida or a statewide association of pharmacists.

106 – b

The pharmacist manager should make 2 backup tapes/disks of drug inventory and prescription information if the pharmacy will be closed or evacuated due to a hurricane or other national emergency.

107 – d

Inventory of controlled substances must be completed at least once every 2 years.

108 – b

The dispensing of a Schedule II opioid for acute pain is limited to a 3-day supply. If specified as medically necessary, this can be extended.

109 – e

A pharmacist registered as a dispensing practitioner can order and dispense up to a 34-day supply of the approved medications under Florida Administrative Code 64B16-27.220 unless there is another quantity or day supply limit specified.

110 – d

An internet pharmacy in the state of Florida must be open for a minimum of 6 days per week.

111 – d

A negative formulary is created by the Board of Pharmacy and Board of Medicine to demonstrate medicinal drugs that should not be substituted with one another due to inequivalence and the potential to cause adverse effects or harm.

112 – e

A prescriber who authorizes an emergency oral prescription for a Schedule II controlled substance must deliver the original written prescription to the pharmacy within seven days of authorizing the oral prescription. The pharmacist must notify the DEA if the prescriber does not deliver the written prescription.

113 – a, c

On the day of a pharmacy closing, the permittee of the closing pharmacy must deliver prescription files to a different pharmacy that is close in proximity and must put a sign on the front entrance advising the public as to which pharmacy the prescriptions were taken.

The permittee of a closing pharmacy must notify the Board of Pharmacy of the closure and notify them of where the prescriptions will be taken before the date of closing. The pharmacy permit should be returned to the Board within 10 days after the pharmacy has closed.

114 – d

The pharmacists serving on the Board of Pharmacy must have been engaged in pharmacy practice in the state of Florida for at least 4 years before appointment to the Board.

115 – c

Florida State Health Online Tracking System (SHOTS) is a statewide online immunization registry that helps keep immunization records. Pharmacists must report immunizations administered to the registry.

116 – c

After three years of inspections with no disciplinary actions, it can be inspected once every two years.

117– d

Pharmacists must practice nuclear pharmacy for at least 1080 hours in the past 7 years in another jurisdiction in order to practice nuclear pharmacy in Florida without meeting the didactic and experiential requirements in the last 7 years.

118 – c

Schedule II controlled substances may be partially dispensed for a terminally ill LTCF patient. Partial dispensing for other patients may only happen if the pharmacist is unable to fill the entire quantity at the time of dispensing.

119 – e

Prescribers suspected to be involved in controlled substance diversion should be reported to the Department of Health and the Drug Enforcement Agency.

120 – b

A pharmacy or pharmacist engaged in sterile compounding may supervise up to three registered pharmacy technicians, or a ratio of 1:3 (pharmacist:technicians).

121 – a

During the first year of operation, the pharmacy must be inspected twice. It may be inspected a minimum of one time yearly after the first year.

122 – d

At a non-dispensing pharmacy where no sterile compounding takes place, a pharmacist can supervise up to eight registered pharmacy technicians at one time, or a ratio of 1:8 (pharmacist:technicians).

123 – e

In order to be registered in the state of Florida as a non-resident pharmacy, the pharmacy must be available to be reached by a toll-free telephone number for a minimum of 40 hours per week.

124 – c

A Medicaid audit of a pharmacy may not take place during the first 5 days of any month because of the typical high volume of workload.

125 – a

Medications are considered misbranded when they are taken from the prescription bottle they were dispensed in and placed into a unit dose container.

126 – e

To be licensed as a consultant pharmacist, a person must hold a license as a pharmacist which is active and in good standing, and successfully complete a consultant pharmacist course of no fewer than twenty hours.

127 – b

The Board of Pharmacy must be notified by the pharmacy department manager when there is a theft or significant loss of a controlled substance.

128 – a

Theft or loss of a controlled substance must be reported to the Board of Pharmacy within one day after discovering such theft or loss.

129 – c

Controlled drugs in this type of pharmacy must be stocked in unit size not to exceed 100 dosage units unless an exception is granted by the Board of Pharmacy.

130 – d

A pharmacist's meal break must not take more than 30 minutes when they are the only pharmacist on duty. If a meal break is longer than 30 minutes, the pharmacy must close until the pharmacist returns.

131 – d

Records must be maintained which provide the name, initials, or identification code of each person who performed a processing function for every medication order. They must be readily retrievable for at least the past four years.

132 – a

Only pharmacists may have the keys or other means to access the prescription department.

133 – e

A prescription copy may be issued to the patient, patient's caregiver, or the patient's prescriber. A prescription copy is not the same as a prescription transfer. A copy is for informational purposes only. If the patient authorizes that a pharmacist at another pharmacy have a copy of a prescription, then it can be done. However, medications cannot be dispensed based on a prescription copy.

134 – c

Pharmacies must back up data from their data processing system at least once a week (every seven days) to prevent data from being lost due to system failure.

135 – b, c, d, e

A written prescription for a medicinal drug must be legibly printed or typed so as to be capable of being understood by the pharmacist filling the prescription; must contain the name of the prescribing practitioner, the name and strength of the drug prescribed, the quantity of the drug prescribed, and the directions for use of the drug; must be dated; and must be signed by the prescribing practitioner on the day when issued.

136 – a

A foreign pharmacy graduate must be supervised at a ratio of 1 pharmacist to 1 intern.

137 – b

A Medicaid audit may not cover a period of time of more than one calendar year. For example, if a Medicaid audit was taking place on July 16th, then records could only be audited between July 16th of the current year and July 16th of the previous year.

138 – a, b, e

Modified Class II institutional pharmacies are typically short-term or primary care treatment centers. These can include: alcoholism treatment centers, rapid in/out surgical centers, correctional institutions, free-standing emergency rooms, and specific county health programs. These types of pharmacies provide specialized pharmacy services that are not typically obtainable from other types of pharmacies.

139 – e

If the Governor issues an emergency order or proclamation of a state of emergency, the pharmacist may dispense up to a 30-day supply in the areas or counties affected by the order or proclamation. However, this does not apply to Schedule II drugs.

140 – c

The consultant pharmacist of record for Modified Class II institutional pharmacies must provide on-site consultations at least once a month.

141 – d

The license renewal date for community pharmacists is September 30th.

142 – a

A prescription department manager may be the manager at only one pharmacy unless otherwise approved by the Board of Pharmacy.

143 – a, b, c, e

Alprazolam, Eszopiclone, Lorazepam, and Zaleplon are Schedule IV medications. Testosterone is a Schedule III medication.

144 – d

Hard-copy printouts of prescription data must contain all of the following: patient name, prescriber name, drug name, drug strength, quantity dispensed, prescription number, date of dispensing, and initials or identification code of the dispensing pharmacist.

The number of refills remaining is not needed. Additional information is needed if the information is not readily retrievable from the computer display.

145 – b

An inspection must be done at least once a year for a pharmacy that does not pass inspections during the first two years or was disciplined. This must be done for at least three years with passing inspections before it can be done less than annually.

146 – e

The controlled substances "Caution" warning, stating that it is a crime to transfer the drug, is required on the label for all controlled substances in the state of Florida. Federally, it is required on the label of Schedule II–IV controlled substances, but not Schedule V.

147 – b

The pharmacy permit renewal date every two years is on February 28th. Permits that are not renewed by this date become null and void after 6 months if not renewed.

148 – d

Pharmacy permits are renewed every two years.

149 – e

A pharmacist must complete a total of at least 200 hours of didactic instruction from an accredited college of pharmacy and supervised practical experience in nuclear pharmacy in order to become licensed as a nuclear pharmacist.

150 – c

A closed drug delivery system is where medications are maintained by the facility and not the patient.

151 – b

Type "A" Modified Class II institutional pharmacies cannot have more than fifteen medicinal drugs on formulary.

152 – e

Prescriptions for Schedule II controlled substances for terminally ill LTCF patients may be partially dispensed for up to 60 days after the issue of the prescription.

153 – d

A pharmacy or pharmacist not engaged in sterile compounding may supervise up to six registered pharmacy technicians, or a ratio of 1:6 (pharmacist:technician).

154 – c

A daily hard-copy printout should be produced within 72 hours of the date of dispensing and should be kept on file in the pharmacy. Individual pharmacists that dispensed that day must sign the document.

155 – a, c, d

A Schedule II prescription can be faxed when the drugs will be compounded for direct administration to a patient, for patients residing in a long-term care facility, or patients enrolled in a hospice care program certified and/or paid for by Medicare.

156 – d

The daily hard-copy printout must be signed by each pharmacist that participated in dispensing or refilling medications on the date of dispensing, and this must be done within 7 days of that date.

157 – a

If using a log book to maintain record of each pharmacist dispensing on a particular day and verifying the information entered into the system was reviewed and was correct, the pharmacists need to sign the log book the day of dispensing.

158 – e

Medication labels from unit dose systems must contain the patient name, prescriber name, prescription number, directions for use, and the Medication Administration Record (MAR). If serving inpatients, it must also contain the vendor pharmacy name.

159 – d

A pharmacist holding a nuclear pharmacist license must complete an additional twenty-four hours of approved coursework every two years that is related to radiopharmaceutical theory, advances in drugs or radiopharmaceutical technology, recent principles of radiation safety, nuclear pharmacy management, or effective communication skills in a multi-disciplinary nuclear pharmacy environment. Twelve hours must be completed each year for a total of twenty-four every 2 years.

160 – a

A pharmacist must obtain at least one hour of continuing education on HIV/AIDS before the first license renewal. The course must include modes of transmission, precautions, infection control, epidemiology of the disease, related infections, management, prevention, testing and confidentiality, reporting, and offering testing.

161 – d

The dispensing of a Schedule II opioid for acute pain is limited to a 3-day supply. If specified as medically necessary, this can be extended to a 7-day supply by the prescriber.

162 – b, c, d

Schedule II-IV controlled substance prescriptions must have a written and numerical notation of the quantity prescribed. Non-controlled medications and Schedule V controlled substance prescriptions are not required to contain both written and numerical notation of the quantity. Schedule I controlled substances are not legal.

163 – e

The license renewal date for consultant pharmacists is December 31st.

164 – b

A pharmacist must complete at least 500 hours of supervised practice experience in nuclear pharmacy, along with 200 hours of didactic instruction in nuclear pharmacy, in order to become licensed as a nuclear pharmacist.

165 – a, b, c, e

The pharmacy must affix a label to any compounded drug that is provided for office use. The label must include: the name, address, and phone number of the compounding pharmacy; the name and strength of the preparation and a list of active ingredients and strengths; the pharmacy's lot number and beyond-use-date; the quantity or amount in the container; the appropriate ancillary instructions such as storage instructions, cautionary statements, or hazardous drug warning labels where appropriate; and the statement "For Institutional or Office Use Only – Not for Resale," or if the drug is provided to a veterinarian, the statement "Compounded Drug."

166 – b

The members of the Drug Wholesale Advisory Council serve a term of 4 years.

167 – d

A pharmacy wanting to centralize certain controlled substance records in a single location must notify the DEA in writing at least 14 days before doing so.

168 – d

A pharmacist must complete a 20-hour continuing education certification program for vaccine administration in order to become certified to administer.

169 – e

Pharmacist signature log books for dispensing record verification must be kept on file for a period of at least four years after the date of dispensing.

170 – d

A log of the sale of Schedule V OTC products must be kept for a period of at least 2 years from the date of sale.

171 – a

Class I pharmacies are those in which all medicinal drugs are administered from individual prescription containers to the individual patient and in which medicinal drugs are not dispensed on the premises. Class II pharmacies employ a pharmacist who provides dispensing and consulting services on the premises to patients of that institution, for use on the premises. Modified Class II pharmacies are short-term, primary care treatment centers. Class III pharmacies are affiliated with a hospital that provide the same services as Class II.

172 – a

Oral controlled substance prescriptions must be reduced to writing immediately.

173 – a, e

If controlled substances are dispensed by a practitioner in the legal course of his/her practice, they must have a label containing: the practitioner's name, patient's name, date of dispensing, directions for use, and the drug name and strength.

174 – e

A Medicaid audit report must be delivered to the pharmacist within 90 days after the conclusion of the audit. A final report should be delivered within 6 months after receiving the preliminary report or final appeal.

175 – d

The owner of the community pharmacy and the new prescription department manager must notify the Board when there is a change in prescription department manager.

176 – a, b, d, e

Paper prescriptions for controlled substances must be written with ink or indelible pencil, typewriter, or printed on a computer printer, and they must be manually signed by the practitioner. A computer-generated prescription that is printed out or faxed by the practitioner must be manually signed.

177 – a

Dispensers are required to report controlled substance dispensing to the E-FORCSE Florida Prescription Drug Monitoring Program via PMP Clearinghouse. Reporting must be done through their electronic system as soon as possible, but no later than the close of the next business day after the day the controlled substance is dispensed.

178 – d

Loss of information from a data processing system in a pharmacy must be reported to the Board of Pharmacy within 10 days of discovering the loss.

179 – a, c, d

A pharmacist must record that a prescription was partially filled, the partial quantity dispensed, and the date of dispensing the partial quantity when dispensing a partial prescription for a Schedule II controlled substance.

180 – d

Pharmacies located outside of the state of Florida that deliver prescriptions to residents of Florida in any manner must be registered with the state of Florida. Non-resident pharmacies must notify the Florida Board of Pharmacy within 30 days of a change in location of the pharmacy.

181 – a, b, d

The negative formulary is for medications that have been determined to not demonstrate significant biological or therapeutic equivalence and should not be substituted. The Board has determined these medications may cause harm or lack equivalent benefit if substituted.

These drugs include: dicumarol, digitoxin, chlorpromazine (solid oral form), conjugated estrogen, pancrelipase (oral forms), and theophylline (controlled release).

182 – e

The immediate inner container label of a radiopharmaceutical to be distributed must be labeled with: the standard radiation symbol; the words "Caution Radioactive Material"; the radionuclide; the chemical form; and the prescription order number of the radiopharmaceutical.

The name of the patient or the words "Physician's Use Only" is one of the labeling requirements for the immediate outer container shield.

183 – d

Modified Class II Type A and B pharmacies may store drugs in bulk, whereas Type C pharmacies may not and must be in patient-specific form.

184 – b

A certified optometrist who has completed a 20-hour board-approved course may prescribe the oral ocular pharmaceutical agents which are listed in the statutory formulary. They may prescribe topical ocular pharmaceutical agents without completing a course.

185 – c

An individual must be at least 18 years or older to purchase pseudoephedrine-containing products in the state of Florida.

186 – c

The Board of Pharmacy must be notified by the transferor pharmacy when ownership of medications is being transferred to a new owner.

187 – b

A nursing home consultant pharmacist must review documents of controlled substance destruction at least once every month to ensure compliance.

188 – b

Nurse practitioners prescribing Schedule II controlled substances may prescribe up to a 7-day supply.

189 – c

Pharmacists must complete 30 hours of continuing education during every 2-year license period before renewal. For a certified pharmacist immunizer, at least 3 hours of the 30 must be related to safe and effective vaccine administration.

190 – b

A pharmacy in Florida must be open for a minimum of 5 days and 20 hours per week.

191 – c

The PDMP (E-FORCSE) must be consulted each time a controlled substance prescription is dispensed for any individual 16 years or older.

192 – e

Under no circumstances may prescription drugs, pharmaceuticals or devices which bear upon the container an expiration or beyond use date which has been reached be sold or dispensed to the public. Accordingly, all outdated, damaged, deteriorated, misbranded, or adulterated prescription drugs and pharmaceuticals shall be removed or quarantined from active stock.

193 – b, e

Counterfeit resistant prescription pads must be used by the following practitioners for all written controlled substance prescriptions: allopathic prescribing practitioners (MD), osteopathic prescribing practitioners (OS), podiatric prescribing practitioners (PO), dentists (DMD or DDS), optometrists (DO), physician assistants (PA), and advanced practice registered nurses (APRN). They are only required for controlled substances, although there is no prohibition from using them for non-controlled substance prescribing. Veterinarians are not required to use them.

Counterfeit-proof prescription pads or blanks may only be purchased from vendors that have been approved by the Florida Department of Health. Pre-printed license numbers are not required. The practitioner's DEA number can be pre-printed on the pads or a space can be provided for their DEA number to be handwritten.

194 – e

A hard copy printout of controlled substances dispensed must be produced within 72 hours of a law enforcement officer requesting such records. These may only be given to a law enforcement officer whose role it is to enforce controlled substance laws.

195 – d

Hard copy printouts of controlled substances dispensed must cover the past 60 days when printed for law enforcement officers.

196 – a

Prescriber information required on a prescription includes: name, profession/credentials, signature, address, zip code, and phone number. Patient information required on a prescription includes: name, address, and age or date of birth. Other information required includes: date of issuance, drug name, strength, quantity, dosage form, and directions.

197 – d

CQI committee summarization records must be kept for a period of at least 4 years.

198 – a

Community pharmacy inspections are carried out by persons from the Department of Health.

199 – b

Redistribution (transfer) of controlled substances may not exceed five percent of the total number of all controlled substances dispensed by a pharmacy during the 12-month DEA registration period.

200 – d

Non-resident pharmacies sending prescriptions to Florida residents must disclose the location, names, and titles of all pharmacists dispensing medications to Florida residents annually.

Contact Us

Pharmacy Testing Solutions is committed to publishing high-quality, accurate test prep materials. We have had multiple pharmacists review this material as well as a copyeditor. However, despite our best efforts, we realize that an occasional error may occur. If you encounter anything that appears to be incorrect, please contact us!

We will immediately review the issue and publish a correction if necessary. This will help to ensure that our content is 100% accurate for future students. And we will also send you a nice reward for any significant errors that are brought to our attention. You may contact us at: PharmacyTestingSolutions@gmail.com.

Thanks for choosing our MPJE review book!

Made in United States
Orlando, FL
21 March 2025